Flesh and Blood

Perspectives on the Problem
of Circumcision
in Contemporary Society

Flesh and Blood

Perspectives on the Problem of Circumcision in Contemporary Society

Edited by

George C. Denniston
University of Washington
Seattle, Washington

Frederick Mansfield Hodges
Yale University
New Haven, Connecticut

and

Marilyn Fayre Milos
National Organization of Circumcision Information Resource Centers
San Anselmo, California

Kluwer Academic / Plenum Publishers
New York, Boston, Dordrecht, London, Moscow

Proceedings of the Seventh International Symposium on Human Rights and Modern Society:
Advancing Human Dignity and the Legal Right to Bodily Integrity in the 21st Century,
held April 4–7, 2002, in Washington, DC

ISBN: 0-306-48333-5

©2004 Kluwer Academic/Plenum Publishers, New York
233 Spring Street, New York, New York 10013

http://www.wkap.nl

10 9 8 7 6 5 4 3 2 1

A C.I.P. record for this book is available from the Library of Congress.

Dedication

This book is dedicated to James Leigh Snyder, MD, FACS, Past President of the Virginia Urologic Society, for his courageous and compassionate commitment to human rights, medical ethics, respect for children, and human dignity.

Preface

Who owns your sex organs? Different cultures today and in different epochs have given a variety of answers to this question. It may seem self-evident that every individual owns and has sovereignty over his or her own body parts, such as the head, legs, nose, stomach, pancreas, and other body parts. The sex organs, however, seem to be an exception. Even though they are as much an integral part of the individual as a leg or a liver, the sex organs are unique in that many cultures have established laws and taboos over the use and even the mere display of the sex organs. Thus, certain cultures have placed constraints over the individual's ownership of his or her sex organs and actively regulate and restrict the individual's access and use of those organs.

In other cultures, the question of ownership of the sex organs is more decisively answered. In any culture where circumcision to any degree of either the male or female is practiced, permitted, encouraged, or even merely tolerated, it is clear that the individual is not considered to own his own sex organs. In the United States today, the medical establishment has created an environment where it is considered acceptable and desirable that anyone for any reason can authorize or execute the amputation of the foreskin from a male child's penis. As a result, millions of American males have been forced to live their lives without ever knowing what it is like to have intact genitalia. At present, 1.2 million American baby boys are subjected to the routine confiscation and destruction of their normal and healthy penile foreskin. This is a body part and a means of experiencing the world that they are not allowed to have.

The majority of Americans involved in this practice either as perpetrators, enablers, or targets have been persuaded to believe that males have no right to keep their sex organs intact. Furthermore, they have been conditioned to accept the underlying belief that a male's sex organs belong not to him but to his parents, to the medical establishment, or to the community as a whole. Even though the male is only legally under the jurisdiction of his parents until the age of eighteen in the United States, elements working within the medical profession have fostered a climate in which it is made to seem normal that parents have the right to make permanent surgical alterations and reductions to the sex organs of the male child that will endure beyond the age of eighteen and remain with him for the duration of his life. Thus, it is the community rather than the individual who exerts absolute control and authority over the sex organs of the individual male.

Analogs for this situation exist in different cultures, but, ironically, not among those Western nations that share a common culture and history with the United States. In Europe, for instance, the circumcision of native European children is almost unimaginable, although Europeans have generally turned a blind eye to the circumcision of those children of immigrants, aliens, and guest workers from foreign countries where circumcision is widely practiced.

The closest analogs for the American situation are to be found among those third-world and middle-eastern cultures with strong histories of theocratic rule, patriarchy, slavery, and religious primitivism. Muslim, Jewish, and certain African tribal cultures make no secret of the fact that they consider the sex organs of the male, and, in many cases also the female, to be public property, to be disposed of according to the dictates of religious hierarchies or in accord with amorphous concepts of tradition that seem impossible to resist. Moreover, these cultures have developed elaborate public rituals and ceremonies in which the target male or female is submitted to the confiscation of parts of his or her sex organs. Thus, it is made patently obvious to everyone in the community that individuals do not own their own sex organs and that the community may take them away without regard to the feelings and intentions of the individual.

For those societies that practice it, deliberate wounding of the flesh and sex organs and the ritualized shedding of genital blood potently advertise the claim to power of the rulers over the ruled. As Sigmund Freud surmised, circumcision is a substitute for the blood ritual of human sacrifice. Indeed, it is a partial human sacrifice. Whether the sex organs of innocent children are sacrificed to appease a deity or to show submission to medical authority, the element of domination, submission, and powerlessness of the individual is the same.

Prevalence, frequency, or ancient origins of this or any other practice, however, do not confer legitimacy or innocuousness. Claims of medical necessity, benefits, or harmlessness are made today by the perpetrators of circumcision for the simple reason that medicine and science are considered to be all powerful and beyond the ability of the layman to question. In those traditionally theocratic cultures where circumcision is incorporated into religious ideologies and mythologies, the claim that circumcision is commanded by supernatural forces may once have been sufficient to stupefy and silence the public into acquiescence, but even in these cultures today, medical mythologies have usurped much of the power that religion once possessed to validate the authority and actions of the rulers. Circumcision perpetrators who were once shaman, witchdoctors, village barbers, and mohels may have been transformed into medical doctors; they may no longer speak the language of religion and instead have learned the language of science; they may no longer claim to be the agents of supernatural forces and instead now claim to represent medical science; and they may no longer insist that circumcision is urgently required and mandated by a fearful deity and now insist that circumcision is urgently required by medical necessity. Nevertheless, the underlying psychosexual motivation to seize and lay claim to the sex organs of others, to wound their flesh and shed their blood, remains, just as irresistible for those who are compelled to control and dominate.

The American Academy of Pediatrics, for instance, has adopted the position that female circumcision should be opposed because it "has no medical benefits."[1] On the other hand, male circumcision, they imply, should not be opposed because they have declared it to have *potential* medical benefits. The unethical nature of this type of reasoning seems beyond the ability of the medical profession as an institution to appreciate. Based on this argument, it could be deduced that female circumcision would be acceptable if doctors were motivated to claim medical benefits for it. Thus, the claim of "medical benefits" has merely replaced the older validating formula of "religious benefits." A genuine ethical assessment would produce the principle that both male and female circumcision are unethical and unacceptable because they violate the individual's right to sovereignty over his or her own body. Even if there were significant medical benefits to male and female circumcision, it would still be unethical to inflict genital reduction surgery on individuals who have neither consented to the surgery nor been given all the objective facts about all the consequences of the loss of these body parts.

It could be argued that medical benefits would accrue with the amputation of almost any body part. An amputated breast would never get cancer or develop infections or require any hygienic care. Leg amputation would have the benefit of reducing the rate of broken legs, stubbed toes, athletes' foot, sprained ankles, and eliminate the need for daily washing. As humorous or ridiculous as this reasoning is when applied to other body parts, it is the same reasoning that is used to justify male circumcision in the United States and female circumcision in those cultures that practice it. The claim of medical benefits is a ruse calculated to deceive, coerce, and pacify. Obviously, given the prevalence of these sorts of uncivilized motivations, both medicine and religion are in need of reform.

The history of most world cultures is marked by a slow but steady progress toward enlightenment and social justice and away from barbarism. Relics of barbarism, however, remain. The process of civilizing even the most civilized cultures is far from complete as demonstrated by the primitive state of medical ethics, or, better stated, as demonstrated by the ability of the medical establishment to ignore ethical pronouncements and mandates.

The contributors to this volume were among those who assembled at Georgetown University in Washington, DC, for the Seventh International Symposium on Human Rights and Modern Society, from 4 to 7 April 2002. The speakers and attendees focused on the vulnerability of human society to medical, economic, and historical pressures that compromise and damage bioethics and the right to sovereignty over one's own body. The speakers provided a much-needed, thoughtful, and detailed analysis of the impact of circumcision on human rights and the development of the concept of bodily integrity. In this last sense, the challenge posed by the contemporary cultural disregard for the individual's right to control his or her own body and sexual destiny serves as a vivid example of how medicine has played a decisive role in shaping and defining cultural attitudes towards male sexuality and the male body.

The contributors to this volume are leading experts in their respective fields. The papers in this book examine the problem of male and female circumcision from a variety of original angles. With a problem as complex and deep-rooted as circumcision, a multiplicity of approaches is required to bring clarity and suggest a way forward.

We look forward to the day when our society will value *life* over a cold, calculating, and corrupt "science" that employs any pretense to divest individuals of their rights and to violate their bodily integrity. The contributors to this volume call upon the people of the world to reject the sly and empty promises of those who would sacrifice our freedoms on the blood-splattered altars of pseudo-science. Circumcision may not always kill the child, but it always and intentionally kills *part* of the child. As such, circumcision is a deliberate destruction and desecration of human life. History has shown that a civilized society cannot support the systematic devaluation of human life for any reason. Instead of being ruled by superstition, fear, greed, and oppression, a civilized society must be guided by reason, courage, and compassion. We are pledged to work for the creation of just such a society.

George C. Denniston

Frederick Mansfield Hodges

Marilyn Fayre Milos

REFERENCE

1. American Academy of Pediatrics. Just the facts. . . circumcision.   URL: http://www.aap.org/mrt/factscir.htm [access date: 24 September 2003]

Acknowledgments

To the people who helped make the Seventh International Symposium on Human Rights and Modern Society, held at Georgetown University in Washington DC, a success, we extend our heartfelt thanks. Special thanks are owed to Ken Brierley, Sheila Curran, Chelo Jacob, and Dr. Peter Ball. In addition, we would like to express our appreciation to the contributors for allowing us to publish their work. We would also like to express our deepest gratitude to Dr. James L. Snyder for his tireless enthusiasm, encouragement, generosity, and friendship. His sage counsel and support have been instrumental in seeing this book project through to completion.

Contents

Chapter 1

BODILY INTEGRITY IN THE BIOTECH ERA
Placing Human Rights and Medical Ethics in Historical Context

Frederick Mansfield Hodges, D.Phil (Oxon)
Department of History, Yale University

Abstract: This paper outlines biotechnology developments that impinge on human rights. I show that the failure of the biotechnology revolution to yield greater human rights protections and instead to consolidate preexisting institutionalized abuses is due in part to the entrance of these abuses into the mainstream prior to the advent and implementation of civil rights and ethical and legal protections. To remedy this situation, the paper suggests strategies for reform so that the right to bodily integrity receives broader social and political support.

Key words: Biotechnology, informed consent, medical experimentation, circumcision, human rights, medical ethics

1.   INTRODUCTION

The way that mothers and newborn babies are processed in the medico-industrial hospital system of the United States has long been influenced by traditions and routines that are based on theories of prominent and vocal doctors rather than on genuinely scientific or humanitarian principles. Efforts to encourage doctors to abandon their invalidated practices have invariably been met with stiff resistance, especially when the required changes would result in greater protections for the right to bodily integrity. When confronted with the fierce opposition that the medical profession has mounted in the face of rising popular resistance to the systematic infliction of circumcision, one is forced to ask the following question: Would the protection of every male's right to bodily integrity result in changes in our society that some people do not want? If so, what do the architects and

Flesh and Blood, Edited by Denniston et al.
Kluwer Academic/Plenum Publishers, New York 2004

perpetrators of this organized and systematized assault on male bodily integrity imagine that they stand to lose? To answer that question, we need to examine the recent history of the progressive social movement for bodily integrity.

It was nearly twenty years ago that Marilyn Milos and Sheila Curran founded the National Organization of Circumcision Information Resource Centers. Through that organization, they reached out to the medical profession, to parents, and to concerned individuals to provide them with accurate information about human genital anatomy, physiology, and its rational care. While they discussed the many benefits and advantages that would result from respecting natural human anatomy in both the hospital and home setting, they also warned of the dangers that can and do result from a disrespect of human anatomy and, of course, of human rights and human dignity. Among other things, they asked the medical profession to examine its own peer-reviewed published literature that conclusively *proved* the harm and inutility of circumcision. They also encouraged the profession to implement these findings into clinical practice.

Instituting reforms in medical practice has always been a problem about finding ways to encourage doctors and hospitals to apply into clinical practice the revolutionary scientific information that they themselves have generated. The notion that circumcision is necessary for any number of medical and social reasons, or the belief that circumcision, at the very least, is innocuous, has had enormous vogue, although the evidence to support it has been thoroughly invalidated. Doctors who are familiar with the relevant medical literature know this. Thus, we must pose the question: What forces are preventing doctors from putting a halt to the practice of systematic circumcision of the newborn? The standard answers that take into account issues of power, money, and face-saving are all correct, but they are not the whole story. There is a new factor that is pushing human rights to the bottom of corporate medicine's priority list.

2.   THE BIOTECHNOLOLOGY REVOLUTION AND THE COMMODIFICATION OF THE FORESKIN

In recent years, the new biotechnology revolution, instead of providing greater incentives for respecting human dignity, has provided the medical industry with additional inducements for maintaining antiquated hospital routines that were established in the 1950s. Additionally, the new technologies spawned by the biotechnology revolution have intensified rather than decreased the medical industry's propensities to view the human body as a rich source of marketable commodities to be used for research and industry. In other words, the medical profession has commodified the human body. For instance, in many if not most hospitals in the US, prospective patients are denied treatment unless they sign a document stating that they understand that the hospital or its agents can and will use any bodily fluids or tissues removed from the patient for "research" purposes unrelated to the patient's treatment regimen.

Furthermore, while the American medico-industrial complex garners an estimated \$2.1 billion a year through the imposition and enforcement of the systematic, assembly-line process of routine circumcision,[1] no one prior to the development of the new biotechnology had predicted that the brave new world of test tube babies, in vitro fertilization, rental of surrogate wombs, fabrication of human organs, xenotransplantation, genetic engineering, and human gene therapy would foster not only the survival of routine circumcision but also its entrenchment as an industrial process, seemingly necessary for the procurement of essential biomaterials to be used for many of the key industrial products of the new technology.

On the one hand, the possibility of commercial harvesting and exploitation of human embryonic stem cells has indeed generated a storm of controversy. Ironically, though, the ongoing commercial harvesting and exploitation of human *foreskin* cells has not yet generated the same level of public and political protest. Why is this? Stem cells are a type of generalized cell harvested from the five-day-old blastocyst that has not yet attached itself to the uterine wall. Foreskin fibroblasts derive from living flesh harvested from human babies after they have exited the womb. By what process of ethical deduction has society decided that the five-day-old blastocyst has a greater right to legal protection than a newborn baby boy?

This moral enigma is partially explained by the fact that stem cell harvesting is a new technology developed in an era in which human rights concerns have gained in ascendancy among the public and independent watchdog groups. Circumcision, however, is a relic from primitive times and alien places where the concept of human rights was nonexistent. Even though medicalized circumcision is a relatively recent phenomenon, it too is a product of a nineteenth-century world where human slavery, child labor, and the political and legal subjugation of women were accepted as normal, necessary, and innocuous. Although the idea that humans beings have human rights had already been beautifully expressed in the French revolutionary *Déclaration de Droits de l'Homme et du Citoyen* [Declaration of the Rights of Man], the American revolutionary *Declaration of Independence*, the *United States Constitution*, and the *Bill of Rights*, American society evidently failed to consider that these rights also applied to children and to all peoples regardless of race, class, age, or ethnicity. Even the Cold War phenomenon of systematic, indiscriminate, industrialized "routine" circumcision of male newborns was brought into production during a time when African Americans were legally disenfranchised, prevented by law enforcement agencies from voting, denied their civil rights, and barred from equal access to governmental services — even though they also paid taxes at the same rate as those privileged enough to enjoy access to those services. As a holdover that had been institutionalized in less enlightened times, routine circumcision has slipped under the modern net of ethical scrutiny. The professionally orchestrated prevalence and the deliberately engineered illusion of banality that shroud circumcision have been allowed to blunt the nation's sensitivities to what would otherwise be an obvious and crude breach of medical ethics.

Nationwide, with 1.2 million American baby boys circumcised each year, circumcisers are collecting between $145,200,000 and $360,000,000 on an annual basis. Factoring in all of the related "hidden" hospital and physician charges resulting from the procedure, as well as the cost of hospitalization, legal fees, multi-million-dollar lawsuit settlements, and surgical reconstruction fees generated to repair the frequent complications, the cost of routine circumcision to insurers and parents in the United States is substantially higher.

One hidden factor that raises the cost of circumcision to the healthcare industry is the additional cost of the hospital stay after circumcision. Between 1990 and 1991, researchers discovered that the difference in hospital length of stay between newborn boys who leave the hospital genitally intact and those who end up being circumcised amounts to an annual cost of $234 million to $527 million *beyond* the charges for the procedure itself.[2]

HCIA-Sachs reports that the total cost of an in-hospital non-therapeutic neonatal circumcision in the United States has risen from $1,154 in 1992 to $1,869 in 1999, a cost increase of sixty-two percent. The total cost of neonatal circumcisions performed in hospitals in the United States was reported to be $2.1 billion in 1999.[3] Even if the various motivations of individual advocates and practitioners of mass circumcision are unrelated to financial gain, it is clear that mass circumcision is highly profitable.

For decades, hospitals and circumcisers were content merely to cut off the foreskins of boys and discard them as medical waste. Now, however, due in part to advances in the biotechnology industry, human foreskins are in great demand for any number of commercial enterprises. Consequently, the marketing of purloined baby foreskins has ballooned into a multi-billion-dollar-a-year industry. The human foreskin has been commodified and traded on the open market without the permission or knowledge of the majority of Americans.

Since the 1980s, shrewd private hospital administrators have realized the enormous profit potential in selling severed foreskins to private bio-research corporations and pharmaceutical companies that require fresh human flesh as raw research material. Hospitals are also in the business of selling foreskins to trans-national biotechnology corporations, such as Advanced Tissue Sciences,[4] Organogenesis,[5] BioSurface Technology,[6] Genzyme, and Ortec International, who use human foreskins as the raw materials for a type of breathable bandage. These corporate giants have emerged to reap enormous corporate profits from the sale of marketable products made from covertly harvested human foreskins. In 1996 alone, Advanced Tissue Sciences could boast about a healthy $663.9 million market capitalization performance.[7]

Pharmaceutical companies use human foreskins in the manufacture of interferon and other drugs, while corporate researchers use them for a wide range of experiments as they search for new profit horizons. International biotech corporations are procuring cells from amputated foreskins and experimenting with artificial skin. Products like LifeCell Corporation's AlloDerm(R) or Advanced Tissue Sciences' Dermagraft-TC, which sells for about $3,000 per square foot, are grown from the unique cells in infant foreskins and used as a temporary wound covering. One foreskin contains enough epithelial regenerative capacity to grow 250,000 square feet of "skin."

According to a report in *Forbes* magazine, the annual market for baby penis-derived products could be $1 billion to $2 billion.[8] Advanced Tissue Sciences has sold about $1 million worth of cultured foreskin products to Proctor & Gamble, Helene Curtis, and other such businesses for pre-market testing. Advanced Tissue Science's foreskin-derived merchandise held a $32 million stock offering in the beginning of 1992.

To further underscore the fact that circumcision has become a goldmine for the medical industry, biotechnology firms like Organogenesis have received suspect fast-track approval from the Food and Drug Administration (FDA) for foreskin-based GraftskinTM. American citizens, doctors, medico-legal experts, and bioethicists were denied the opportunity to request a full hearing over the ethics of the trafficking and marketing of living human sex organs that have been harvested for this purpose without the permission or knowledge of the "donor."9 In January 1998, when an FDA committee was formed to review Advanced Tissue Sciences' application for approval of its baby foreskin-derived product, Dermagraft, they gave a respected human rights attorney only five minutes to address the committee to point out the legal and ethical problems with the harvesting and marketing of living body parts without consent or financial compensation. On 26 May, 1998, the FDA granted approval for what amounts to legalized penile plunder.[10]

In his investigation of this legalized trafficking in human body parts, John A. Erickson put the following pertinent questions to the CEO of a major pharmaceutical company that purchases baby foreskins for experimentation:

How much does one infant foreskin sell for?

How many foreskins have been sold?

Who sells them? Doctors? Midwives? Mohels? Hospitals?

Who buys them?

Are there any middlemen, and if so, who are they?

Are the foreskins sold per foreskin or by weight?

Do circumcisers have a financial incentive to cut off as much skin as possible?

Is a foreskin still marketable if it has been covered with or injected with anesthetic? Do circumcisers have a financial incentive not to use an anesthetic?

Are some types of foreskin more in demand than others? (White, Black, Latino, Asian?)

Are parents told that their baby's foreskin will be sold? Are they asked if their baby's foreskin may be sold?

Who is the legal owner of a baby's foreskin after it has been cut off?

Who is the legal owner of a baby's foreskin before it is cut off?

Is it ethical to cut off a baby's foreskin, charge his parents for the operation, sell his foreskin without telling his parents, and keep the money? Is it legal?

Are the foreskins of children and adults being sold too?

Are other parts of people's bodies being cut off — or out — and sold without their knowledge or consent?

If someone cuts part of another person's body off — or out — and sells it without obtaining signed legal consent from the person cut, and the person who buys it makes money from it, who does that money rightfully belong to?

The CEO of this company never replied to Mr. Erickson's letter.

As they become even more profit-driven, hospitals should come under closer scrutiny for the kinds of bargains they strike with biotechnology corporations. One must seriously question the claim of independence and objectivity of physicians on hospital payrolls who advocate routine newborn circumcision. One may well ask whether the anti-foreskin "studies" generated by circumcision advocates are actually little more than the self-serving green lights that corporate hospitals and biotechnology firms need to proceed with their agenda of turning living babies' body parts into cash.

Given the egregiousness and brutality of this situation, it is worth considering whether such medico-industrial practices are exceptional or whether they are merely part of a pattern of traditional abuses of human rights.

3.   THE AMERICAN MEDICAL ASSOCIATION IN CONFRONTATION WITH THE NUREMBERG CODE AND THE DECLARATION OF HELSINKI

After World War II, following the revelations of the shocking medical experiments that were inflicted by Nazi doctors on concentration camp prisoners, concerned lawyers formulated the *Nuremberg Code for Permissible Human Experiments*, an exemplary and enlightened document that stands as the first and the most thorough attempt to restrain doctors from interfering with people without informed consent. Seeking to shore up the loopholes in the *Nuremberg Code*, the newly formed World Medical Association soon thereafter worked diligently to establish an additional ethical code that would serve as a guide to doctors, particularly in hospitals, who tried to add to the sum of medical knowledge by experimenting on the patients under their care.

Even after the German medical profession had been disgraced through its association with the military experiments in concentration camps, world-wide public uneasiness about investigations that continued to be carried out in hospitals threatened to disgrace the medical professions in the United States and Britain. As a response to this situation, The World Medical Associations' *Draft Code of Ethics on Human Experimentation*, which was unveiled in 1962,[11] was remarkable for its insistence that the very groups targeted for experimentation by Nazi doctors should be guaranteed special protections from use, misuse, and abuse by doctors. Accordingly, it stipulated that prisoners and children or anyone incapable of giving consent because of age, mental incapacity, or of being in a position in which they are incapable of exercising the power of free choice, should not be used as subjects for experimentation.

The American medical profession, represented by the American Medical Association (AMA), strongly disagreed with these protections, arguing that consent was irrelevant. At first, the American medical elite completely ignored the *Draft Code of Ethics*. Although it was published in European medical journals, not a single American journal published the *Draft Code of Ethics* or even acknowledged its existence. Still, American medical leaders were very worried that this document might actually be ratified. In 1958, the AMA convened a special council to draw up a statement on experimentation in man and informed consent. The final report fiercely defended the doctor's "right" to perform experiments on what it called "civil prisoners," a group that the AMA defined as including "inmates of orphanages and asylums for the insane as well as prisoners in jail."[12] Evidently, to be an orphan was equivalent to being a criminal without any legal protection against compulsory medical experimentation.

The AMA report also attacked the concept of *informed consent*, complaining that "explicit observance of point one [informed consent] would require detailed explanation to the participating subject with the inevitable result that he would become self-conscious and introspective."[13] The AMA report further insisted that it was unnecessary to provide information to subjects about risk "when *innocuous* procedures are undertaken"[14] [italics added]. It is evidently no accident that advocates for mass circumcision have always expended great effort to characterize circumcision as "innocuous."

The AMA report made a special point of attacking the first point of the *Nuremberg Code*, which states: "The voluntary consent of the human subject is absolutely essential."[15] The AMA complained that "a rigid interpretation of this would effectively cripple, if not eliminate, most research in the field of mental disease...."[16] Significantly, the AMA attempted to reconcile this first point with the observation that, since "mental cases" could be likened to children in an ethical and legal sense, it was sufficient for the doctor to solicit consent from the child's guardian.[17]

This is the only reference to children in the AMA report, but it is highly significant, for it clearly implies that children have no legal standing, that their consent is unnecessary, that doctors are free to do whatever they like to them as long as they call it "innocuous," and that doctors can solicit "proxy content" from the child's guardians. Of course, this stance was technically unnecessary since routine circumcision in the 1950s almost always was performed without the parents' consent or knowledge. It is likely, though, that the AMA saw the smoke on the horizon and tried to devise a legal shelter before the firestorm of public demand for informed consent swept over them.

When the AMA realized that the suppression of information about the World Medical Association's *Draft Code* was not going to stop this august body from continuing its work to ratify the *Code*, the AMA swiftly moved to infiltrate and take over the World Medical Association in order to gut the *Draft Code of Ethics* of its most important clauses — those that protected children and prisoners. The takeover was swift and complete. By 1964, the AMA had maneuvered itself into being the sole financial supporter of the World Medical Association, and the president of the AMA, Dr. Edward Annis, was now conveniently installed as the president of the World Medical Association.

In June 1964, at the World Medical Assembly held in Helsinki, the finalized code of ethics was ratified and given the name by which it is now known: *The Declaration of Helsinki.*[18] Although this version was superficially identical to the previously published draft code, all references to informed consent and to bans against using children or prisoners had been silently excised. In fact, there was no reference to children at all. Thanks to American pressures, the document that was originally intended to protect children and prisoners from medical experimentation ended up protecting no one except doctors. In the United States, the *Declaration of Helsinki* was warmly welcomed, but in Europe, it was uniformly condemned.

4. AMERICAN MEDICAL EXPERIMENTS ON CHILDREN

While it is tempting to speculate that forces within the AMA were determined to weaken the *Declaration of Helsinki* and purge it of the dangerous idea that "children should not be the subject of human experiment" in order to place the nationwide experiment of mass circumcision beyond legal or ethical scrutiny, the full picture is even grimmer An editorial in the *British Medical Journal* angrily suggested that, if the *Helsinki Code* had been passed intact and free of American interference, a series of horrible American medical experiments on children that had just come to light could never have occurred. What were these experiments?

Europeans were shocked at a paper that was published in 1964 in the *New England Journal of Medicine,* detailing the results of an experiment that took place in Boston in which eighteen children who had undergone corrective heart surgery were simultaneously and secretly subjected to an additional series of surgical ordeals that recalled the horrors of the Nazi doctors' experiments at Auschwitz.[19] Without their own or their parents' consent or knowledge, and for reasons unrelated to their heart condition and without any possible medical benefit to the children, surgeons completely removed the thymus gland from eleven of the children, and, in seven, who unwittingly served as "controls," doctors took only a biopsy of the thymus. Then, a full-thickness skin homograft was sutured in place on the chest wall.

The experimenters claimed that they were interested in determining whether thymectomy affected the survival of skin grafts.

It is important to emphasize that information gleaned from this experiment on thymectomy was irrelevant to the problems of corrective heart surgery. The children were chosen opportunistically because they just happened to be undergoing chest surgery. Their healthy thymus glands were destroyed, and their chests were mutilated and scarred by a skin graft they did not need. Defending the experiment and attacking the call for a code of ethics to protect children from this sort of medical abuse, Joseph Garland, the editor of the journal carped: "A blind adherence to an inflexible code may be unrealistic…"[20] Garland paid lip service to the *Nuremberg Code*, but seemed to argue that it did not apply to American doctors because it was too rigid and did not bend to "the nuances of modern research."[21] The American medical profession seemed to believe that the *Nuremberg Code* was little more than a formal condemnation of the Nazis rather than an ethical guide that American doctors were supposed to follow.

Europeans were horrified again when news of yet another objectionable Nazi-like American medical experiment was made public.[22] In this case, doctors targeted perfectly normal and healthy newborn infants who had the misfortune to have been born to women who were incarcerated in a state reformatory. Doctors secretly fed the babies live poliovirus in their bottles so they could determine whether there was a hereditary resistance to the crippling disease.

There exist many other documented proofs of the American medical profession's traditional devaluation of children. At the very least, these cases indicate that the physician's human obligations to his patients are sometimes abused. Most significantly, however, these cases effectively convey the professional atmosphere of the time in which routine circumcision was imposed on the citizens of the United States. Subjecting healthy newborn baby boys to penile reduction surgery and unjustifiably exposing them to risk without absolute and immediate medical necessity is merely one of the many lapses from a cultivated sense of ethics that has been endemic to American medicine throughout its history.

Consequently, none of the important ethical codes under discussion seem to have had any restraining effect on American doctors who are unable to understand the difference between guinea-pigs and human beings, especially when they are young or collected together in penitentiaries, reformatories, orphanages, or other institutions. Indeed, the American medical profession seems to have regarded the maternity hospital as a veritable institution of correction. Anyone who ventured or emerged inside was subjected to medical correction because they were regarded as having no right to object, refuse, or discontinue compulsory treatment. Hence, in such a climate, it was deemed perfectly legitimate for American doctors to devalue the lives of children, to experiment upon them, and to inflict surgical amputations at the doctor's own discretion or whim.

5.   EXACTLY *WHO* FEELS THREATENED BY HUMAN RIGHTS?

Considering the historical context in which routine circumcision was systematically inflicted on the citizens of the United States during the Cold War era, one may again question what circumcisers fear most about human rights, especially the right to bodily integrity.

Despite the enormous profits that would be lost by the protection of males from circumcision, it can be convincingly argued that circumcisers are more concerned that the demise of the circumcision industry would signal the loss of their power to control the ideologies that govern our culture. Distinct from the motivations and agendas of individual circumcision advocates, on an aggregate industrial level, the primary driving force behind mass circumcision remains an anti-male ideology that has traditionally served to answer the ambition of the American medical profession to maintain control and authority over the sexual organs of the male. The proof of this observation is to be found in the history of medicalized circumcision, which was introduced in the nineteenth century and most widely inflicted on American boys as a means of preventing, "curing," and punishing masturbating.

When sex surgery becomes punishment or even a means of controlling sexual expression, in a very real political sense, the medical profession can been seen as utilizing circumcision as an instrument of political violence and repression. Whether used from the 1870s to the 1960s as a means of making masturbation unsatisfying or functionally impossible (a mistaken but fervently held doctrine that runs through the medical literature) or whether used today to micromanage the individual's sexual behavior ostensibly to prevent AIDS, in infliction of involuntary circumcision is about control, repression, and domination.

The American medical profession's historic insistence that it has the right to determine the level of sexual pleasure that a male will be permitted to experience during his lifetime and the accompanying claim that the medical profession has the right to regulate and restrict, through circumcision, the private use of the sex organs attests to this history of active repression. I would argue that the intentional imposition of a massive, permanently disfiguring wound on the penis and the infliction of severe pain through penile surgery (frequently and traditionally performed without any type of anesthesia or analgesia) is an act of violence intended to terrorize the victim as much as to intimidate adult witnesses and to impress upon them the "fact" that the medical profession has declared ownership of the sexual organs of the male and has absolute jurisdiction over their fate. Such motivations are difficult to defend. The biotechnological reliance upon harvested foreskins for industrial success, however, has furnished a politically expedient and rationalization for mass circumcision that is easier to defend in public debate in the current economic and political climate.

Even though the primary targets of this institutional violence are today more likely to be newborn infants, the screams of the baby are just as powerful and soul-destroying, if not more so, to the indirect victims composed of the audience of parents and other members of the population. Furthermore, the male who has been processed through this system of sexual disempowerment is left with a permanent physical reminder of his subjugation to medical authoritarianism. His remnant flesh has been impressed with the self-serving medical doctrine that the male body is inherently flawed and degenerate in its natural, unprocessed state. The artificiality and both the anatomical and functional limitations of the circumcised penis grimly illustrate the current self-serving medical ethics doctrines currently promoted by circumcision advices that no male has the right to keep his body intact, that anyone for any reason may with impunity deprive a male of part of his sexual anatomy, and that no male has the right to experience any higher, richer, more varied, or broader level of sexual sensations than the bare minimum necessary to trigger procreative ejaculation. In other words, the American medical profession has adopted the profoundly unethical, unjust, and chilling attitude that no male owns his own penis. The infliction of foreskin amputation signals that the medical profession can and will impose anatomical and functional limitations on male sexuality. Hence, circumcision solidifies the profession's control over sexuality in a permanent and brutal way.

Most Americans remain blithely ignorant of these ethical problems. Even when the issue is highlighted for them, Americans have been conditioned to dismiss these ethical concerns as "alarmist," "unpatriotic," and "unrealistic." The conventional wisdom among most doctors working in the field is that there is little need to examine the ethical implications of what they are doing to our children's bodies. Circumcisers market their activities as "services" that are either medically indicated or socially demanded. They disguise their campaign to amputate the foreskin from little boys' penises behind convenient and misleading rhetoric about "the parents' right to choose circumcision for their son."[23] The lay public is never told that the alleged social demand for infant circumcision is a classic example of "supply-led demand." Parents request or acquiesce to physician pressure to authorize the surgical removal of part of their child's penis because parents have been conditioned through exposure to a lifetime of pro-circumcision marketing campaigns to make this request. Sadly, the leaders in the medical community, the media, the government, and the business community, with a few notable exceptions, remain as reluctant today as they were a generation ago to engage in a broad public debate over what must surely be the most radical, problematic, and widespread experiment ever carried out by industrialized medicine. As such, circumcision is a chilling product of a coldly menacing, soulless science.

Genuine medico-legal ethics will always clash with the self-serving pseudo-ethics charades hatched by the anti-foreskin militants and their supporters who have established a beachhead in the medical profession and even in the field of ethics.[24] True ethical principles, however, neatly harmonize with established doctrines of human rights that are supported by nearly all non-aligned, non-partisan international ethics committees. An authentic formulation of medical ethics is never, to any degree, compromised by feeble attempts at cultural relativism or eroded by exceptions based on claims of "public health," "tradition," "culture," "heritage," or special dispensation because of claims of victim status.

6.   CONCLUSION

As I have tried to show here, the perpetrators of medical abuse have shown themselves incapable of restraining their compulsions and acting with compassion towards their "subjects" by simply leaving them alone. Rather than fostering an evaluation of the ethical implications of its approach to the human body, the biotechnology revolution instead has solidified and intensified the medical profession's traditional predacious, managerial, autocratic, and dehumanizing approach to human beings.

A happy and mutually enriching marriage between human rights and scientific progress must certainly be possible. At present, however, the medical industry has shown little interest in purging itself of an unscientific ideology whose lineage can be traced back to the age of barbarism.

The problem lies not with biotechnology in the abstract but with its practitioners, whose attitudes have been shaped and constrained by the imperious and brutalizing American medical culture that has prevailed over the last few centuries. In an industrialized medical environment with a strong history of disregarding the human right to autonomy and sovereignty, the opportunities for authentic bioethics to shape the course of biotechnology are limited. More specifically, in a medical culture that continues to insist that males have no right to maintain sovereignty, control, or even possession of their own genital body parts, it has proven difficult for biotechnologists to resist the temptation to join in the plunder and lay claim to the biological commodities and cellular byproducts generated by the circumcision industry.

Self-styled ethicists who are psychologically or psychosexually blinded, enthralled, or employed by the biotechnology and circumcision industries may devise clever ethical-sounding ruses designed to maintain the status quo, but, in the end, history will be the final judge of the ethical content of their actions. It seems clear that any rhetorical or ethical formulations that supports rather than condemns the commodification of the human body, the deliberate wounding of a healthy child's body, the destruction of normal human anatomy and functionality to any degree, and even the slightest violation of bodily integrity and sovereignty are deceitful, fraudulent, and, ultimately will be correctly seen as criminally liable.

REFERENCES

1. Bollinger D. Intact versus circumcised: male neonatal genital ratio in the United States. Circumcision Reference Library. 13 November 2000.
URL: http://www.cirp.org/library/statistics/bollinger3/
2. Mansfield CJ, Hueston WJ, Rudy M. Neonatal circumcision: associated factors and length of hospital stay. J Fam Pract 1995 Oct;41(4):370-6.
3. Bollinger D. Intact versus circumcised: male neonatal genital ratio in the United States. Circumcision Reference Library. 13 November 2000.
URL: http://www.cirp.org/library/statistics/bollinger3/
4. Manson B. Forget pork bellies, now it's foreskins. San Diego Reader (4 1995): pp. 12, 14.
5. Brewer S. New skin twin life- and look-save. Longevity (September 1992): p. 18.
6. Rosenberg R. Companies see $1.5b market in replacement skin products. Boston Globe (19 October 1992): pp. 22-3.
7. Hall CT. Biotech's big discovery. San Francisco Chronicle. (25 October 1996): pp. E1, E4.
8. Pitta J. Biosynthetics. Forbes (10 May 1993): pp. 170-1.
9. Arnst C. Science and Technology. The latest from the labs: human skin: the FDA is about to approve commercial use of living tissue grown by two biotech outfits. Business Week (18 May 1998): pp. 118-22.
10. Reuters (29 May 1998).
11. World Medical Association. Draft Code of Ethics on Human Experimentation. BMJ 1962 Oct 27;2(5312):1119.
12. Council on drugs, Beecher HK. Experimentation in man. JAMA 1959 Jan 31;169(5):461-78. [here, p. 465.]
13. Council on drugs, Beecher HK. Experimentation in man. JAMA 1959 Jan 31;169(5):461-78. [here, p. 472.]
14. Council on drugs, Beecher HK. Experimentation in man. JAMA 1959 Jan 31;169(5):461-78. [here, p. 464.]
15. Council on drugs, Beecher HK. Experimentation in man. JAMA 1959 Jan 31;169(5):461-78. [here, p. 472.]
16. Council on drugs, Beecher HK. Experimentation in man. JAMA 1959 Jan 31;169(5):461-78. [here, p. 472.]

17. Quotation from A.C. Ivy, chief medical consultant to the War Crimes Trials. In: Ivy AC. History and ethics of use of human subject in medical experiments. Science 1948 Jul 2;108:1-5. cited in: Council on drugs, Beecher HK. Experimentation in man. JAMA 1959 Jan 31;169(5):461-78. [here, p. 472.]

18. Declaration of Helsinki: Human Experimentation: Code of Ethics of the World Medical Association. BMJ 177.

19. Zollinger RM Jr, Lindem MC Jr, Filler RM, Corson JM, Wilson RE. Effect of thymectomy on skin-homograft survival in children. N Engl J Med 1964 Apr 2;270(14):707-10.

20. Garland J. The ethics of human experimentation. N Engl J Med 1964 May 7;270(19):1014-5.

21. Garland J. The ethics of human experimentation. N Engl J Med 1964 May 7;270(19):1014-5.

22. Experimental medicine. BMJ 1962 Oct 27;2(5312):1108-9. [here, p. 1108.]

23. For classic examples of sham ethics designed to shield circumcisers and circumcising groups from legal scrutiny and public protest, see: Benatar M, Benatar D. Between Prophylaxis and Child Abuse: The Ethics of Neonatal Male Circumcision. Am J Bioeth. 2003 Spring;3(2):35-48. Also, see: Batzer FR, Hurwitz JM. Male Neonatal Circumcision: Ritual or Public-Health Imperative. Am J Bioeth. 2003 Spring;3(2):1-2.

Chapter 2

AN ANALYSIS OF THE ACCURACY OF THE PRESENTATION OF THE HUMAN PENIS IN ANATOMICAL SOURCE MATERIALS

Gary L. Harryman, MA

Coordinator, National Organization of Restoring Men, Southern California Chapter (NORM-SoCal)

Abstract: The purpose of this study is to identify and analyze the accuracy of the anatomical source materials regarding the human penis that are immediately available to medical school students and medical professionals. Ninety sources were vetted for entries and images of the penis – definitions, photos, illustrations, and drawings. We find 67% of the depictions of the human penis are anatomically incorrect. Of the primary images of the human penis, 71% are incorrect, while 54% of the secondary are incorrect. It is evident that the penis is misrepresented in the medical literature used in medical schools. The penis is routinely defined and depicted in a partially amputated condition, as if this were a natural state, without explanation or caveat. This study indicates that students are being misinformed about fundamental anatomy.

Key words: Medical education, penis, foreskin, prepuce, circumcision

1.   INTRODUCTION

The purpose of this study is to identify and analyze the accuracy of the anatomical source materials regarding the human penis that are immediately available to medical school students and medical professionals. Section 2 describes the sources that were analyzed. Section 3.1 presents our principal (numerical) findings (percentages of correct and incorrect presentations of the penis/foreskin), while section 3.2 includes a number of individual observations. Section 4 includes a discussion of what our findings tell us about the way circumcision is perceived and dealt with in the medical profession, and the consequences thereof for the professional and the public.

2.   SOURCES

The source materials on which this study is based are those available to medical students and medical professionals in five Los Angeles, California college campus bookstores and two biomedical libraries.[1] The source materials include medical textbooks, life-sized medical models, medical study aids, medical charts, medical dictionaries, medical encyclopedias, medical catalogues, and (medical) general interest books; the findings hereinafter referred to as entries and images.

Ninety (90) sources were vetted for entries and images of the human penis – definitions, photos, illustrations, and drawings.[2]

3.   FINDINGS

3.1   Principal Findings

In the 90 sources, we found three hundred sixty-five (365) images of the penis. Of these 365 images, one hundred twenty-two (122), 33%, showed anatomically correct depictions of the foreskin, while two hundred forty-three (243), 67%, showed penises from which the foreskin had been amputated. Of those 243 disfigured images, only one includes an explanation of why the foreskin was absent.[3]

When the primary images (which present the penis as the direct subject of study or discussion) and secondary images (which show the penis incidental to an image of another organ, e.g. the bladder or the hip joint), are distinguished and separated, we find that primary images are more often incorrect than secondary images. Out of two hundred seventy-two (272) primary images of the penis, only seventy-nine (79), 29%, were anatomically correct in their depiction of the foreskin. One hundred ninety-three (193), 71%, were anatomically incorrect (i.e. foreskin absent) in their depiction of the foreskin. Out of ninety-three (93) secondary images of the penis,[4] forty-three (43), 46%, were anatomically correct in their depiction of the foreskin. Fifty (50), 54%, were anatomically incorrect in their depiction of the foreskin.

Approximately half of the anatomically correct primary and secondary images appeared in only five of the 90 sources.[5]

Only one source identified a disfigured image of a penis without a foreskin as having been "circumcised."[6] Not one source mentioned the erogenous functions of the foreskin. None illustrated or explained the kinematics of the gliding function of the foreskin, its contribution to human sexuality, and its value to both sexes. Not one source illustrated, identified, labeled, or explained the structure and/or function of the primary neurological feature of the foreskin system, and perhaps of the penis – the ridged band.[7]

3.2   Concurrent and Incidental Observations

The glossaries of all the sources were also vetted for the entries "foreskin" and "prepuce." In all but four of those sources,[8] typically the definitions for foreskin and/or prepuce included the tag line: "... is the part that is removed at circumcision." This clearly indicates an underlying prejudice. One source identified the image of a natural penis as "uncircumcised."[9] Another stated that the glans of "an uncircumcised penis" is covered by the prepuce.[10] We know of no other human organ that is literally defined by medical professionals as something that is "unamputated."

One dictionary did not have an entry or illustration for penis, foreskin, prepuce, or ridged band. It did have an entry for circumcision.[11]

Only one source attempted to accurately explain the lack of foreskin with an arrow to the circumcision scar line labeled "remains" of the foreskin.[12]

Typically, illustrations had lines or arrows running from a label to the anatomical feature the label described. Nine sources had illustrations showing the penis with foreskin intact but not labeled as were the other anatomical features.[13] One source had two sectional illustrations of the penis in which the label identifying the foreskin did not point to the foreskin, but pointed to the glans or the preputial space.[14]

Three sources included illustrations depicting the penis without foreskin, but nonetheless with labels for the foreskin pointing to the glans.[15]

One illustration of the penis depicted the foreskin as being the same thickness as the glans.[16] Another depicted the foreskin as nearly as thick as the penis shaft.

Only six of the 90 sources had images depicting the natural, commonplace akroposthion condition wherein the puckering foreskin extends beyond the tip of the glans (The classic image depicted in virtually all visual art, worldwide, before twentieth century American art.).[17] In two of those six sources the label under the photo was the pejorative epithet "phimosis;" apparently misrepresenting a natural and benign human condition as pathological.[18]

One definition of the word prepuce was accompanied by an illustration of a natural penis labeled "redundant."[19]

In one definition of the word foreskin, the source repeated a three-hundred-year-old myth that smegma is "secreted by Tyson's glands."[20]

Most of the sources authored and published outside the U.S. accurately depicted the natural condition of the penis.[21]

One source claims to be based on the reputable National Library of Medicine's "Visible Human Project."[22] Its liner notes state: "anatomically exact and complete" and to "recreate visually the exact forms of the body and all its parts." The book has no images of the penis with foreskin. The words foreskin, prepuce, and ridged band are not in its index or glossary.

Where possible, every source was also vetted for images of the vulva and/or clitoris. Every one of them depicted the female genitalia accurately and anatomically intact.

In this research we also have noticed that, of the books that mention the foreskin, those published before 1970 were usually correct in their descriptions and illustrations, while those published between 1980 and 1996 are almost universally incorrect. Books published in the last five years tend to be increasingly mixed.

4.   DISCUSSION

When we tally the evidence, we find 71% of the primary images and 67% of the total primary and secondary depictions of the human penis in recently published sources that are readily available to medical professionals and students are anatomically incorrect (i.e. foreskin is absent). In addition, as shown by our incidental observations, the inaccurate presentation of the penis not only involves the absence of the foreskin, but also instances of blatantly inaccurate presentations. Based on these findings, we must conclude that the penis is an organ that is grossly misrepresented in the medical literature used in medical schools. The penis is routinely defined and depicted in a partially amputated condition, without explanation or caveat. To presume the foreskin-less images depicted in the literature all resulted from observed natural conditions defies credibility — the incidence of aposthia is rarer than 1:400 births. Therefore, a reasonable person would conclude that virtually all of the images of penises without foreskins would have to represent unidentified surgical amputations.

Authors of the depictions of the foreskin in both the medical and popular literature apparently suffer from a form of unconscious self-censorship or are deliberately misrepresenting facts. Medical students and the public at large are being misinformed on the form and function as well as the fundamental value of the natural human penis. Any explanation brings up questions of ethics and violations of implied social contract between authors and readers, publishers and buyers, doctors and patients.

Science is dependent upon objectivity and clarity of knowledge. The evidence we found indicates that anatomy books used in medical schools in the U.S. cannot be trusted to accurately depict the human body, and medical dictionaries and encyclopedias cannot be trusted to truthfully define, describe, and illustrate the natural human condition. By logical extension this raises questions about whether a U.S.-educated doctor's judgment about related matters can be trusted, and whether the public should be warned to question the quality of care U.S. medical school graduates can provide.

This study shows that medical students are being misinformed about fundamental male anatomy. While the female genitalia are invariably represented accurately in the anatomical literature, male genitalia are not. Misrepresenting the absence of the human foreskin as trivial or congenital normalizes the mutilated image of the circumcised penis. This may explain why female circumcision is commonly perceived as radical sexual surgery, but the loss of the entire foreskin system of the penis is characterized as irrelevant by powerfully repeated visual and verbal implication; its unique kinematics not worthy of mention, its value not worthy of comment, and the concentrated innervation of its ridged band unworthy of safeguarding.

5.   CONCLUSION

Our findings indicate that foreskin amputation of males in the U.S. has degenerated to the status of medical dogma rather than appropriate science. Such widespread distortion of fundamental and obvious anatomical truths indicates the diagnostic objectivity and therapeutic credibility of physicians educated in the U.S. deserves careful scrutiny. Absent profession-wide re-education, the ethical and legal consequences of their actions regarding male anatomy, may justifiably be criticized in what was already a perilously unstable legal environment for physicians. Indeed, as one physician recently warned: "...the legal system may no longer be able to ignore the conflict between the practice of circumcision and the legal and ethical duties of medical specialists."[23]

REFERENCES

1. Research was carried out in the medical lecture classrooms, labs, campus bookstores and libraries of the University of California, Los Angeles (UCLA), the University of Southern California (USC), and Santa Monica College (SMC).

2. The 90 sources include:

Abrahams PH, Hutchings RT, Marks SC Jr. McMinn's Colour Atlas of Human Anatomy. 4th ed. London: Mosby; 1998. p. 232.

Bickley LS. Bate's Guide to Physical Examination and History Taking. 7th ed. Philadelphia: Lippincott Williams & Wilkins; 1999. p. 387.

Blackbourne LH, Antevil J, Moore Ch. Anatomy Recall. Philadelphia: Lippincott Williams & Wilkins; 2000. p. 270, 279.

Budget Functional Francis Torso. Skokie (IL): Anatomical Chart Company; 2002.

Caime KW, Garfinkel P, et al. The Male Body: An Owners Manual. St. Martin's Press; 1996.

Clayman C, editor. The Human Body. London: Dorling Kindersley Publishers; 1995. p. 184.

Clayman CB, editor. AMA Encyclopedia of Medicine. An A-to-Z Reference Guide to over 5,000 medical terms including Symptoms, Diseases, Drugs & Treatments. New York: Random House; 1989. p. 466, 779, 862.

Clemente CD. Anatomy – A Regional Atlas of the Human Body. 4th ed. Philadelphia: Lippincott Williams & Wilkins; 1997. p. 1, 179, 186, 188, 286-7, 290, 302, 308.

Cohen J. The Penis Book. Cologne: Konemann Verlagsgesellschaft MbH; 1999. p. 2-100.

Complete Care Manikin. Skokie (IL): Anatomical Chart Company; 2002.

Cull P, editor. The Sourcebook of Medical Illustration. Parthenon Publishing Group; 1989. p. 164.

Deluxe Condom Training Model. Skokie (IL): Anatomical Chart Company; 2002.

Denoyer-Geppert Multi-Torso. Skokie (IL): Anatomical Chart Company; 2002.

Davies A, Blakely AGH, Kidd C. Human Physiology. Edinburgh: Churchill Livingstone; 2001. p. 628.

Dirckx JH, editor. Stedman's Concise Medical Dictionary for the Health Professions. 3rd ed. Baltimore: Williams & Wilkins; 1997. p. A9, A12, A19-21, PA26.

Dorland's Illustrated Medical Dictionary. 28th ed. Philadelphia: WB Saunders; 1994. p. 1652.

Dorland's Illustrated Medical Dictionary. 29th ed. Philadelphia: WB Saunders; 2000. p. 1780.

Dox I, et al., editors. Melloni's Illustrated Medical Dictionary. 4th ed. London: Parthenon Publishers; 2002. p. 368, 492, 527.

Dulbecco R, editor. Encyclopedia of Human Biology. San Diego: Academic Press; 1991;4. p. 486.

Dulbecco R, editor. Encyclopedia of Human Biology. San Diego: Academic Press; 1991;6. p. 12, 14-5, 562.

Dulbecco R, editor. Encyclopedia of Human Biology. 2nd ed. San Diego: Academic Press; 1997;7. plate 15, 518.

Elliott, Boone. Recent advances in the management of the neurogenic bladder. Urology 2000 Dec Supp l 6A; 56(6A). p. 78.

Gatesville Care Manikin. Skokie (IL): Anatomical Chart Company; 2002.

Gatesville Child Care Manikin. Skokie (IL): Anatomical Chart Company; 2002.

Goldman DR, editor in chief. American College of Physicians. Complete Home Medical Guide. 1st ed. New York: DK Publishing; 1999. p. 707, 709, 713, 717-9, 721-2, 726-7, 763, 771, 810.

Goldstein I. Male Sexual Circuitry. Scientific American 2000 Aug. p. 70-5.

Gosling, et al. Human Anatomy. 2nd ed. London: Gower Medical Publishers; 1990. p. 5.

Gosling, et al. Atlas of Human Anatomy. Philadelphia: JB Lippincott; 1985. p. 5.

Gotto, AM, editor. The Cornell Illustrated Encyclopedia of Health. 1st ed. Washington DC: Lifeline Press; 2002. p. 890.

Harris S, Harris J. Reproductive System. Permachart (cram chart). Concord: Papertech; 1999.

Harris S, Harris J, Permachart Quick Reference Guide–Reproductive System. Concord: Permachart; 1999.

Hatzichristou, Goldstein. Penile Microvascular Arterial Bypass. Surgery Annual. Appleton & Lange; 1993. p. 218.

Hellstrom WJG. Male Infertility & Sexual Dysfunction. New York: Springer; 1997. p. 16, 39.

Jacob S. Anatomy–An Examination Companion. Edinburgh; New York: Churchill Livingstone; 1995. p. 342, 345.

Keeffe EB. Know Your Body. The Atlas of Anatomy. Berkeley: Ulysses Press; 1999. p. 130, 132-3, 135.

Knobil E, Neill JD. Encyclopedia of Reproduction. San Diego: Academic Press; 1998;2. p. 39.

Knobil E, Neill JD. Encyclopedia of Reproduction. San Diego: Academic Press; 1998;3. p. 37, 739-48.

Larsen DE, editor. Mayo Clinic Family Health Book. New York: W. Morrow; 1996. p. 47, 1196, 1209, 1226, 1228.

Lumley JSP. Surface Anatomy. The Anatomical Basis of Clinical Examination. 3rd ed. Edinburgh; New York: Churchill Livingston; 2002. p. 49.

Lutjen-Drecoll E, Rohen JW. Atlas of Anatomy–The Functional Systems of the Human Body. Baltimore: Williams & Wilkins; 1998.

MacPherson G, editor. Black's Medical Dictionary. 38th ed. London: A&C Black; 1995. p. 415.

McCracken TO, general editor. New Atlas of Human Anatomy. MetroBooks; 2000. p. 106-7, 118-9, 148-9, 152-3, 155.

Male Model with Bladder. Skokie (IL): Anatomical Chart Company; 2002.

Male Pelvis Catherterization and Enema Simulator. Skokie (IL): Anatomical Chart Company; 2002.

Male Reproductive System [chart]. Skokie (IL): Anatomical Chart Company; 2002.

Marieb EN, Mallatt J. Human Anatomy. 3rd ed. San Francisco: Benjamin Cummings; 2001. p. 689-90, 702, 704, 709-10.

Martini FH, Bartholomew EF, Bledsoe BE. Anatomy & Physiology for Emergency Care. Parasmus (NJ); Prentice Hall; 2002. p. 17, 532, 554, 569.

Martini FH, Timmons MJ, McKinley MP. Human Anatomy. 3rd ed. Upper Saddle River (NJ): Prentice Hall; 2000. p. 710, 712, 720.

Moore KL, Agur AM. Essential Clinical Anatomy. Baltimore: Lippincott Williams & Wilkins; 1995. p. 183.

Moore KL, Dalley AF. Clinically Oriented Anatomy. 4th ed. Baltimore; Philadelphia: Lippincott Williams & Wilkins; 1999. p. 360, 403, 406-8.

Mosby's Medical, Nursing, and Allied Health Dictionary. 6th ed. St Louis: Mosby; 2002. plate A-37, p. 700.

Netter FH. Atlas of Human Anatomy. 2nd ed. E. Hanover (NJ): Novartis; 1997.

Oliver MV. Rapid Review. Anatomical Reference Guide. Skokie (IL): Anatomical Chart Company; 1996. p. 30.

O'Toole MT, editor. Miller-Keane Encyclopedia & Dictionary of Medicine, Nursing, & Allied Health. 6th ed. Philadelphia: WB Saunders; 1997. plate 13, p. 623.

Paley M. The Book of the Penis. New York: Grove Press; 1999. p. 3, 100-114.

Patient Peevy Manikin. Skokie (IL): Anatomical Chart Company; 2002.

Patton KT, Thibodeau GA. Mosby's Handbook of Anatomy & Physiology. St. Louis: Mosby; 2000. p 546.

Perez V. Quick Study Academic–Male Reproductive System [chart]. Boca Raton (FL): BarCharts Inc; 1999.

Petrou SP, Barrett DM. The Use of Penile Prosthesis in Erectile Dysfunction. Seminars in Urology 1990; 8(2). p. 141, 144-47.

Putz R, Pabst R, editors. Sobotta Atlas of Human Anatomy. 21st ed. Munich: Lippincott Williams & Wilkins; 2000. p. 233, 235, 252.

Putz R, Pabst R, editors, Atlas of Human Anatomy. 13th ed. Philadelphia: Lippincott Williams & Wilkins; 2002;2. p. 214, 231, 233-5, 252.

Raff H. Physiology Secrets–Questions you will be asked in classrooms, on tests, on board exams. Philadelphia: Hanley & Belfus; 1999.

Rhoades R, Pflanzer RG. Human Physiology. 3rd ed. Fort Worth: Saunders College Publishers; 1996. p. 902, 908.

Rohen W, Yokochi C. Color Atlas of Anatomy. Tokyo: Igaku Shoin; 1983. p. 319.

Rohen W, Yokochi C, Lutjen-Drecoll, E. Color Atlas of Anatomy. 4th ed. Baltimore; Philadelphia: Lippincott Williams & Wilkins; 1998. p. 316-7, 323-24, 326-7, 450-1, 453-4.

Rohen W, Yokochi C, Lutjen-Drecoll, E. Color Atlas of Anatomy. 5th ed. Philadelphia: Lippincott Williams & Wilkins; 2002. p. 318, 324, 332-3, 336.

Schlegel, Goldstein. Anatomical Approach to Varicocelectomy. Seminars in Urology 1992;10(4). p. 245.

Schwartz SI, et al., editors. Principles of Surgery. 7th ed. New York: McGraw Hill; 1999. p. 1758.

Seeley RR, Stephens TD, Tate P. Essentials of Anatomy & Physiology. 4th ed. Boston: WCB/McGraw Hill; 2002. p. 523.

Segen JC, The Dictionary of Modern Medicine Illustrated. Parkridge (NJ): Parthenon Publishing Group; 1992. p. 115.

Seidel HM, Ball JW, Dains JE, Benedict GW. Mosby's Guide to Physical Examination. 4th ed. St Louis: Mosby; 1999. p. 645.

Snell RS. Clinical Anatomy for Medical Students. 6th ed. Philadelphia: Lippincott Williams & Wilkins; 2000. p. 359, 367-8.

Snell RS. Clinical Anatomy – An Illustrated Review with Questions and Explanations. Baltimore; Philadelphia: Lippincott Williams & Wilkins; 2000. p. 94.

Spark RF. Sexual Health for Men. The Complete Guide. Cambridge (MA): Perseus Publishing; 2000. p. 39, 310.

Springhouse Atlas of Human Anatomy. Springhouse (PA): Springhouse Corporation; 2001. p. 112, 245-7.

Stedman TL. Stedman's Medical Dictionary. 27th ed. Baltimore: Lippincott, Williams & Wilkins; 2000. plate 26.

Swan R. The Human Body on File. Facts on File; 1983. p. 10.002.

The Urinary Tract [chart]. Skokie (IL): Anatomical Chart Company; 2002.

Thibodeau GA, Patton KT. Structure and Function of the Body. 11th ed. St Louis: Mosby; 2000. p 455.

Thibodeau GA, Patton KT. Anatomy & Physiology, Male Reproductive System. St Louis: Mosby; 1996. p. 11, 996-1013.

Thompson J, Wilson S. Health Assessment for Nursing Practice. St Louis: Mosby; 1996. p. 531-557.

Tortora GJ. Principles of Human Anatomy. 8th ed. New York: John Wiley; 1999. p. 772, 783.

Tortora GJ. Principles of Human Anatomy. 9th ed. New York: John Wiley; 2002. p. 488, 784-5, 795.

Tortora GJ, Tallitsch RB. Anatomy and Physiology with Cat Dissections. 6th ed. Upper Saddle River (NJ): Prentice Hall; 2000. p. 368, 644-5.

Townsend CM, Beauchamp DR, editors. Sabiston Textbook of Surgery: The Biological Basis of Modern Surgical Practice. 16th ed. Philadelphia: WB Saunders; 2001. p. 1682-3.

VanDeGraaff K-M. Human Anatomy. 6th ed. New York: McGraw Hill; 2002. p. 699, 701, 710-1, 715, 720.

Venes D editor. Taber's Cyclopedic Medical Dictionary. 19th ed. Philadelphia: FA Davis; 2001. p. 821, 1607.

Westheimer RK. Sex for Dummies. 2nd ed. Foster City (CA); IDG Books Worldwide; 2001. p. 16-7.

Williams PL. Gray's Anatomy–The Anatomical Basis of Medicine and Surgery. 38th ed. New York: Churchill Livingstone; 1995. p. 352, 1838-9, 1842, 1857.

Willis MC. Medical Terminology: the language of health care. Baltimore: Williams & Wilkins; 1996. p. 434.

3. Thompson J, Wilson S. Health Assessment for Nursing Practice. St Louis: Mosby; 1996. p. 543.

4. Some secondary illustrations were so crudely drawn that it was unclear if the penis was intact or circumcised. Those illustrations were not considered in the figures.

5. Those five sources include: Thompson J, Wilson S. Health Assessment for Nursing Practice. St Louis: Mosby; 1996; Keeffe EB. Know Your Body. The Atlas of Anatomy. Berkeley: Ulysses Press; 1999; Netter FH. Atlas of Human Anatomy. 2nd ed. E. Hanover (NJ): Novartis; 1997; Putz R, Pabst R, editors. Atlas of Human Anatomy. 13th ed. Philadelphia: Lippincott Williams & Wilkins; 2002;2; Tortora GJ. Principles of Human Anatomy. 9th ed. New York: John Wiley; 2002.

6. Thompson J, Wilson S. Health Assessment for Nursing Practice. St Louis: Mosby; 1996. p. 543.

7. For more information about the ridged band, refer to: Taylor JR, Lockwood AP, Taylor AJ. The prepuce; specialized mucosa of the penis and its loss to circumcision. Br J Urol 1996;77:291-5; Taylor J. The prepuce: what, exactly, is removed by circumcision–a preliminary report. Second International Symposium on Circumcision. 30 April-3 May 1991, San Francisco, California; Cold CJ, McGrath KA. Anatomy and histology of the penile and clitoral prepuce in primates: evolutionary perspective of specialised sensory tissue of the external genitalia. In: Denniston GC, Hodges FM, Milos MF, editors. Male and Female Circumcision: Medical, Legal, and Ethical Considerations in Pediatric Practice. New York: Kluwer/Plenum; 1999. p. 19-29; Cold CJ, Taylor JR. The prepuce. BJU Int 1999;83 Suppl 1:34-44; Gollaher DL. Circumcision. A History of the World's Most Controversial Surgery. New York; 2000.

8. The four sources that did not include that line are: Dorland's Illustrated Medical Dictionary. 28th ed. Philadelphia: WB Saunders; 1994; Dorland's Illustrated Medical Dictionary. 29th ed. Philadelphia: WB Saunders; 2000; Dirckx JH, editor. Stedman's Concise Medical Dictionary for the Health Professions. 3rd ed. Baltimore: Williams & Wilkins; 1997; Stedman TL. Stedman's Medical Dictionary. 27th ed. Baltimore: Lippincott Williams & Wilkins; 2000.

9. O'Toole MT, editor. Miller-Keane Encyclopedia & Dictionary of Medicine, Nursing, & Allied Health. 6th ed. Philadelphia: WB Saunders; 1997. p. 623.

10. Tortora GJ. Principles of Human Anatomy. 8th ed. New York: John Wiley; 1999. p. 783.

11. Segen JC. The Dictionary of Modern Medicine Illustrated. Parkridge (NJ): Parthenon Publishing Group; 1992. p. 115.
12. Clayman CB, editor. AMA Encyclopedia of Medicine. An A-to-Z Reference Guide to over 5,000 medical terms including Symptoms, Diseases, Drugs & Treatments. New York: Random House; 1989. p. 466.
13. Thibodeau GA, Patton KT. Anatomy & Physiology, Male Reproductive System. St Louis (MO): Mosby; 1996; Patton KT, Thibodeau GA. Mosby's Handbook of Anatomy & Physiology. St Louis: Mosby; 2000; Thibodeau GA, Patton KT. Structure and Function of the Body. 11th ed. St Louis: Mosby; 2000; Mosby's Medical, Nursing, and Allied Health Dictionary. 6th ed. St Louis: Mosby; 2002. plate A-37; Oliver MV. Rapid Review. Anatomical Reference Guide. Skokie (IL): Anatomical Chart Company; 1996; Rohen W, Yokochi C, Lutjen-Drecoll, E. Color Atlas of Anatomy. 5th ed. Philadelphia: Lippincott Williams & Wilkins; 2002; Snell RS. Clinical Anatomy–An Illustrated Review with Questions and Explanations. Baltimore; Philadelphia: Lippincott Williams & Wilkins; 2000; Clayman C, editor. The Human Body. London: Dorling Kindersley Publishers; 1995; Dox I, et al., editors. Melloni's Illustrated Medical Dictionary. 4th ed. London: Parthenon Publishers; 2002.
14. Clemente CD. Anatomy–A Regional Atlas of the Human Body. 4th ed. Philadelphia: Lippincott Williams & Wilkins; 1997. p. 287, 290.
15. Rohen W, Yokochi Ch. Color Atlas of Anatomy. Tokyo: Igaku Shoin; 1983. p. 319; Clemente CD. Anatomy – A Regional Atlas of the Human Body. 4th ed. Baltimore; Philadelphia: Lippincott Williams & Wilkins; 1997. p. 1, 179, 186, 188, 286, 287, 290, 302, 308; Patton KT, Thibodeau GA. Mosby's Handbook of Anatomy & Physiology. St Louis: Mosby; 2000. p 546.
16. Snell RS. Clinical Anatomy for Medical Students. 6th ed. Philadelphia: Lippincott Williams & Wilkins; 2000. p. 359.
17. Larsen DE, editor. Mayo Clinic Family Health Book. New York: W. Morrow; 1996. p. 1196, 1209; Keeffe EB. Know Your Body. The Atlas of Anatomy. Berkeley: Ulysses Press; 1999. p. 130, 132-3, 135; Thompson J, Wilson S. Health Assessment for Nursing Practice. St Louis: Mosby; 1996. p. 535; Dox I, et al., editors. Melloni's Illustrated Medical Dictionary. 4th ed. London: Parthenon Publishers; 2002. p. 368; Cohen J. The Penis Book. Cologne: Konemann Verlagsgesellschaft MbH; 1999. p. 2-100; Netter FH. Atlas of Human Anatomy. 2nd ed. E. Hanover (NJ): Novartis; 1997.
18. Larsen DE, editor. Mayo Clinic Family Health Book. New York: W. Morrow; 1996. p. 47; Thompson J, Wilson S. Health Assessment for Nursing Practice. St Louis: Mosby; 1996. p. 543.
19. Dox I, et al., editors. Melloni's Illustrated Medical Dictionary. 4th ed. London: Parthenon Publishers; 2002. p. 527.
20. Venes D editor. Taber's Cyclopedic Medical Dictionary. 19th ed. Philadelphia: FA Davis; 2001. p. 821.
21. I.e. Canada, United Kingdom, Germany.
22. McCracken TO, general editor. New Atlas of Human Anatomy. MetroBooks; 2000. p. 106-7, 118-9, 148-9, 152-3, 155, 222, 231.
23. Canning, DA. Informed consent for neonatal circumcision: an ethical and legal conundrum. J Urol 2002; 168 (4 Pt 1):1651.

Chapter 3

THE IMPORTANCE OF THE FORESKIN TO MALE SEXUAL REFLEXES

H.S. Meislahn[1] , BA, MBA, and J.R. Taylor[2], MB, FRCPC
1 .*Director, National Organization of Circumcision Information Resource Centers of Illinois.*
2. *Health Sciences Centre and University of Manitoba, Winnipeg, Manitoba, Canada.*

Abstract: The authors propose that the foreskin is the primary sensory tissue of the penis and that the foreskin's ridged band is built to trigger ejaculation as part of a functional whole that also includes the frenulum, glans, and urethra. The study evolved from research which demonstrated specialized nerve end-organs in the ridged band, and from pre-tests showing that intact subjects are more likely than circumcised subjects to experience reflexes triggered by traction on penile skin, namely, erection of the penis and contraction of the bulbocavernosal muscle. The authors then developed a website which describes the foreskin's anatomy and function and asks intact males whether, in their opinion, the foreskin and its ridged band play an important role in sexual intercourse. The overwhelming majority has firmly agreed, and, for every nine who found the foreskin more important than the glans to sexual intercourse, only five found the glans more important.

Key words: Foreskin, ridged band, penis, anatomy, function, reflexes

1.   PRIOR STUDIES: A CONSISTENT THREAD LEADING TO PRESENT STUDY

The foreskin consists of an outer layer of ordinary skin and an inner layer of specialized junctional mucosa which includes a band of ridged mucosa that encircles the penis, radiating from the frenulum (Figure 1). This ridged band contains a high concentration of Meissner corpuscles, which are a common type of nerve end-organ. The specific location of these end-organs,

Flesh and Blood, Edited by Denniston et al.
Kluwer Academic/Plenum Publishers, New York 2004

27

on the ridged band, was elucidated for the first time by Taylor, Lockwood, and Taylor.[1]

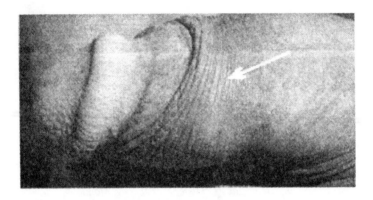

Figure 1. Ridged band
The ridged band is separated from the glans by smooth (non-ridged) mucosa. The arrow points to the boundary between ridged band and true skin of foreskin. Courtesy of Medical Post.

As cited in Taylor, Lockwood, and Taylor, prior studies in microscopic anatomy had clearly established the existence of specialized nerve end-organs in the foreskin. However, none of these studies had located the corpuscles on any specific part of the foreskin nor had any prior anatomist identified or described the ridged band.

Prior research that revealed the foreskin's rich innervation includes an important series by R. K. Winkelmann, MD, a research dermatologist at the Mayo Clinic. In a January 1959 report on preputial innervation, he stated that "The mucocutaneous end-organs extend from the distal margin of the prepuce to the site at which hairy skin begins, where they diminish and disappear."[2] (The term "distal" here refers to the margin at which the retracted foreskin is continuous with the glans.) He further stated: "One primitive [mucocutaneous] ending was found in the prepuces of 30 newborn infants, while many well organized end-organs are present in each sample from the prepuce of the adult."[3] He discussed end-organs of the glans in almost the same terms, stating that "mucocutaneous end-organs are present over the surface of the glans penis, and especially about the coronal sulcus."[4] He had referred in his discussion of the foreskin to the presence of Vater-Pacini corpuscles and found the same corpuscles "in the subcutaneous tissue of the glans in their normal form."[4]

In 1956, Winkelmann had examined the cutaneous innervation of the newborn prepuce, which was the first study focussed specifically on the innervation of the foreskin rather than the innervation of all penile tissue. This report was also the first to publish photo micrographs of nerves in the prepuce, including the Vater-Pacini corpuscle, which is the only form of genital corpuscle ordinarily present in the newborn. Winkelmann observed that the specific form of these corpuscles was highly unusual: "It is apparent in our material that all the bodies present have coiled or serpentine form that is best explained by continued growth in a limited space. The coils occur in relation to large vessels. Such a form lends itself admirably to the perception of changes in pressure and tension in the tissue, as the coils are oriented in three dimensions."[5]

Nor was the 1956 study created in a vacuum. Winkelmann stated that "Probably the first reference to innervation of the prepuce is the notation by Bichat (1801) of the division of the genital nerves into finer branches which lose themselves eventually in the glans penis and the prepuce."[6] Also, "In 1893 Dogiel...found in the inner surface of the prepuce and the frenulum preputii, Meissner corpuscles, genital bodies, and endbulbs."[7] Winkelmann also cited Ohmori (1924): "In a 5 year old boy he found a typical genital body, and then in a 14 year old he found several typical genital bodies....He believed the glans penis and prepuce has the same type innervation because they differentiated from the same mass of cells and had basically the same, rich innervation."[7]

Winkelmann cautioned that none of these earlier studies was supported with photomicrographs and there were significant differences and inconsistencies between them.[7] However, taken in total with Winkelmann's work and Taylor, Lockwood, and Taylor, several conclusions are evident:

1)   None of these studies, extending over two centuries, even hints that the foreskin is poorly innervated.

2)   None suggests that the foreskin is inferior to the glans in degree of innervation.

3)   All the studies subsequent to Bichat identify end-organs in the foreskin, many finding Meissner corpuscles among them.

4)   The most thorough and credible researcher from the past is Winkelmann, because he developed research techniques previously unknown and published extensive photomicrographs of his work. It is also significant that he openly acknowledged how handy it was for his work to have a ready supply of freshly amputated foreskins. There is not a hint anywhere in his writings that he connected the dots between the importance of the foreskin as sensory tissue and a possible breach of

medical ethics in condoning amputation of foreskins from persons incapable of granting informed consent.

In view of this strong chain of evidence, what are we to make of references that misstate and ignore the record we have just examined? They are not hard to find. The American Academy of Pediatrics' 1999 Task Force Report on Circumcision, despite its strengths in some areas, passes quickly over the sexual role of the foreskin, saying only that "One study [Taylor, Lockwood and Taylor] suggests that there may be a concentration of specialized sensory cells in specific ridged areas of the foreskin but not in the skin of the penile shaft."[8-9]

To the contrary, the cited source for this comment did not "suggest" but rather stated as an assertion of fact that "Missing tissue [from the circumcised penis] included a band of ridged mucosa located at the junction of true penile skin with smooth preputial mucosa. The ridged band contains more Meissner's corpuscles than does the smooth mucosa and exhibits features of specialized sensory mucosa."[10]

The AAP's reference to "One study" clearly implies that only one study argued for a concentration of specialized nerve cells in the foreskin. To the contrary, as we have just seen, there were major earlier studies, and these the AAP ignored.

The AAP's failure to focus on circumcision as a loss of sexually important tissue left wide the gate for dismissive and unsupported conclusions by others who claim the mantle of professional authority. For example, the on-line *Harvard Men's Health Watch* for October 2001 stated (before the article was withdrawn) that "There is no reliable evidence to support the claim that newborn circumcision increases the risk of sexual problems in adulthood or that it impairs sexual satisfaction in either partner."[11] It is now time to examine evidence that we have developed showing how the highly innervated foreskin participates in and triggers important male sexual reflexes.

2.   PRELIMINARY TESTS

The presence of specialized nerve endings in the foreskin suggests they serve a sexual purpose. Clues include the following:

1) Form typically follows function, and it therefore seems unlikely that highly concentrated nerve endings in sexual tissue would have no function.

2) For many intact males, the inner layer of the foreskin and its ridged band seem to deploy at the commencement of sexual intercourse so that the ridged band covers the thickest part of the penile shaft and is therefore in close proximity to mucosal tissue in the vagina. Pure coincidence would seem an unlikely explanation for this juxtaposition.

3) It is difficult to argue that the nerve endings are a residual, no longer needed artifact of evolution, because the foreskin is more elaborated in the human than in other primates.[12-13] Far from disappearing, comparative anatomy suggests the opposite.

4) The investigators observed that, in a very small test, the ridged band sometimes takes on a distinct red flush at the peak of erection. This phenomenon does not square well with the thought that the primary purpose of this highly innervated tissue is to serve some other, non-sexual purpose.

These clues pointed to the need for a preliminary test to determine if the ridged band plays an important role in sexual reflexes. A reflex is a response that is involuntary not requiring conscious perception or conscious action from the subject. Focusing on reflexes would therefore lessen subjectivity and possible distortion of results which might occur from looking only at subjects' conscious perceptions, which can be colored by information previously accumulated in the subjects' higher brain centers. Finally, focus on reflexes, some of which can be mediated through the spinal cord without participation by the brain, may take some air out of the often-heard assertion that "sex is all in the brain" so that presence or absence of the foreskin "doesn't really matter."

Our first step was to test whether circumcised and intact men experience the same sexual reflexes. We framed questions for small numbers of volunteers that they could answer with a simple "yes" or "no" based on distinct, observable phenomena. The intention was to show whether the ridged band, which is almost always lost to circumcision, mediates sexual reflexes and especially if its nerve endings are likely to act as stretch receptors. It will be recalled that testing for reflexes caused by stretching is consistent with Winkelmann's 1956 finding that Vater-Pacini corpuscles, which are present not only in the newborn but in adults, is well suited to "the perception of changes in pressure and tension in the tissue."[5] The ridged band as stretch receptor is also consistent with evidence, including a photograph, in Cold and Taylor showing that the sheet of smooth dartos muscle, well known as part of scrotal skin, is also part of the foreskin and of penile shaft skin as well.[14] Because form implies function, the presence of muscle fibers in penile skin implies that the fully retracted foreskin, which would otherwise lie loosely on the shaft, firms up in erection so that the ridged band can respond to stretching anywhere along the penis and thus trigger a stretch reflex.

To test whether the ridged band is important to sexual reflexes, we asked if stretching shaft skin induces erection, which for intact males entailed retracting the foreskin. To test the same reflex in circumcised men, we asked if, when erect, added stretching of shaft skin causes contraction of the bulbocavernosal muscle. To examine the concept of the ridged band as stretch receptor, we asked if penile skin of the erect penis is firmer and tighter than skin when the penis is flaccid.

We also tested the reality of an unexpected sexual reflex, which, when the penis is erect, seems to cause the surface of the penis to take on directionality. Directionality appears to be entirely forward-facing when the foreskin is retracted but may create a retarding effect between the inner foreskin and the glans when the foreskin is covering the glans.

Table 1. Preliminary survey of penile reflexes

Does gentle stretching of shaft skin elicit erection?

	Yes	No
Intact	11	0
Circumcised	5	3

When erect, does added stretching of shaft skin cause contraction of bulbocavernosal muscle?

	Yes	No
Intact	11	0
Circumcised	3	5

Does penile skin shorten and tighten during erection?

	Yes	No
Intact	8	3
Circumcised	3	3

Do you detect forward directionality in penile skin when you are erect?

Intact	8	2
Circumcised	4	4

Both groups of volunteers ranged in age from their early twenties to sixty and over. All were provided written questions and a written description of the relevant anatomy and of the physiological questions we were seeking to study. They were to carry out the tests privately and report their findings principally by e-mail or United States mail. All were guaranteed anonymity.

For reasons of practicality, we had chosen subjects who were knowledgeable about the foreskin. Most circumcised subjects were members of the National Organization of Restoring Men (NORM), though most at the time of the study had reported minimal progress on foreskin restoration. Some intact subjects had actively studied circumcision and had encouraged parents to leave their sons intact. We made no attempt to generate panels of subjects who would be random with respect to any key variables, because we believed that there would be a steep learning curve before subjects could carry out the proposed tests reliably. This learning curve put a premium on knowledge over randomness in sample selection. Also, we accepted small sample size because, at this early stage, our intention was only to determine if preliminary results appeared to warrant a more definitive study.

Our initial decision on subject selection proved sound, because, even with knowledgeable subjects, there were many initial questions. That the subjects were seriously interested in providing reliable results was very beneficial to the results we finally achieved, because, when they had doubts about the meaning of questions as initially worded, they said so. A trial run with the circumcised subjects produced some seemingly implausible responses, especially about directionality, and the investigators therefore provided a videotape showing how to conduct all the tests, as well as re-worded questions. For a few subjects, investigators followed up by telephone to resolve remaining uncertainties.

Results of these preliminary tests encouraged us to undertake a survey that would enlist a much larger group, this time focusing only on intact subjects, and that would provide a thorough, easily understood, and clearly illustrated description of the foreskin and its ridged band. As shown in Table 1, preliminary results that impelled us onward included the finding that retracting penile skin led to erection for intact subjects by eleven to zero. Only five of eight circumcised subjects reported that they became erect when they stretched shaft skin. All eleven intact subjects could feel contraction of the bulbocavernosal muscle (located just behind the scrotum) when they stretched the ridged band during erection, whereas only three of eight circumcised subjects reported this effect when they stretched remaining skin on the shaft of the erect penis. The ridged band as stretch receptor got a boost from the finding that foreskin and shaft skin shortened and tightened during erection for eight of eleven intact subjects. Only three of six circumcised subjects responding to this question detected a tightening and shortening of penile skin when they were erect. With respect to surface directionality during erection, eight of ten intact subjects who answered this question reported forward directionality, compared with four of eight circumcised subjects.

Encouraged by these results, we availed ourselves of a medium of communication that could easily reach and survey intact males around the world: the Internet.

3.   THE RIDGED BAND WEBSITE: OBJECTIVES AND CONTENT

The investigators had several reasons to utilize the worldwide web for a survey of preputial reflexes. The web reaches parts of the world where a much higher percentage of males are intact than in the United States, and it is so widely used that obtaining a large number of responses was feasible. The web also offers privacy, so that men could test our ideas at their own pace without the presence of lab coats and test tubes, which can cause penises to wilt. We also knew that validating tests would be non-invasive and structured for simplicity, so that carrying out the project via the web would be a practical strategy. Finally, the web is a wonderful classroom, and we were confident that the ridged band website would enlighten visitors, whether or not they were candidates for the survey. Many visitors have made use of the site's comment section to obtain answers to their individual concerns about the foreskin.

Pretests had shown that survey subjects are unlikely to provide reliable answers unless they first learn basic information about the anatomy and function of the foreskin and its ridged band. The Ridged Band Website, at http://research.cirp.org, is therefore focused on education, beginning with an abstract summarizing the authors' position. This states: "The foreskin is the primary sensory tissue of the penis," that "the 'ridged band,' a part of the foreskin is built to trigger ejaculation," and that "the ridged band, frenulum, glans and urethra are a functional whole, along with specialized skin of the penile shaft."

The website describes the anatomy of the foreskin in words and pictures. The anatomical text sets forth three basic principles:

1)   Structure and function are closely related so that "If we know what a structure looks like, we can make a reasonable guess at its function."

2)   The foreskin can only be understood as one part of the whole penis.

3)   "[M]ore than any other part of the body...the penis must meet the needs of both user and use."

The text states that the foreskin is double-layered like the lips, that it shares with the scrotum and penile shaft skin a unique feature, namely, a thin sheet of muscle fibers embedded right in the skin, and that the foreskin also has a ridged band of strongly corrugated tissue normally hidden from view just inside the tip of the foreskin, which incorporates large bunches of coiled nerve endings. Photographs illustrate these points.

The website also discusses function: "The functions of the glans and foreskin are similar, and overlapping, but come fully into their own at different times during intercourse." The single statement in the website that produced the most surprise was in the discussion of function: "Compared with the true (outer) skin of the foreskin [which is specialized to detect feather-light touch and other sensations], the glans is only feebly sensitive to light touch, pain, heat and cold." Some respondents questioned this statement but, after self-testing, reported that, sure enough, we were right!

The site's discussion of foreskin function also introduced the idea that the ridged band triggers ejaculation. Adjacent tissues cause it to stretch, and the ridged band is instantly alerted to changes in position of the penis within the vagina by special changes in penile skin, apparent only on erection, which cause it to stiffen and shorten and to take on marked forward directionality.

To help visitors solidify their understanding of the anatomy and function of the foreskin, we repeated much of the information from these sections in captions that accompany the photographs and then in a separate section entitled Frequently Asked Questions (FAQ).

The Ridged Band Website concludes with an invitation for intact adult males to help ongoing research by answering questions about the foreskin and its ridged band. The site provides a questionnaire and also follow-up surveys that went only to those who had responded to the first survey. The first questionnaire focused on whether respondents agreed with broad, basic concepts in the website, and the second primarily tested their agreement with specific, verifiable elements within the over-all concept.

4. THE RIDGED BAND WEBSITE: SURVEY RESULTS

The overwhelming majority of survey participants concurred that information on the website matches their experience as intact adult males, and that descriptions of the anatomy of the foreskin and its ridged band are reasonably accurate. As shown in Table 2, ninety-one percent of the 199 respondents concurred with each of these statements. Nearly as many, eight-eight percent, agreed that the sexual role of the foreskin is similar to that outlined on the website. Eighty percent believed that the ridged band plays an important role in sexual intercourse, and, for every five participants who found the glans more important in sexual intercourse than the foreskin, nine found the foreskin more important. Only thirteen percent felt that the site exaggerates the importance of the foreskin.

Eighty-eight respondents, or forty-four percent, provided comments (reproduced in Table 3). The authors categorized these comments as "analytical/descriptive," "concerned or naive about the foreskin," and "positive or negative feelings about site and/or the foreskin." Many comments touched on more than one category.

Responses have come in steadily for almost a year, from inauguration of the site 13 March 2001, through the cut-off date for the present report on 19 February 2002. Men responding to the survey are of all ages from early adulthood to sixty and over. More than half are younger than forty, and this age distribution reflects typical demographics of the web.

During February 2002, we invited participants in the initial survey to answer additional questions. The primary purpose was to further validate the importance of the foreskin as sexual tissue by encouraging participants to test with their own anatomy the specific sexual reflexes discussed in the website.

Follow-up responses [Table 4] corroborated the reality of the penile reflexes we had described in the website. The great majority of respondents found that stretching the foreskin causes erection, that erect penile skin has forward directionality, and that the skin of the penis is tighter and firmer during erection. A question containing the word "bulbocavernosal" produced many "unsure" responses. We therefore restated the question and added more information. The question as amended produced results consistent with the rest of the survey: The great majority of respondents detected contraction in the muscle just behind the scrotum when they further stretched skin on the shaft of the erect penis.

The follow-up survey also confirmed the broad geographical reach of the survey. About half of respondents live outside the United States.

The great majority reported that their foreskins cover more than half the glans when they are erect. This finding tends to corroborate the foreskin's usefulness for easing vaginal entry and for keeping the glans comfortably covered during nocturnal erections. It suggests yet another way that the penis acts as an interacting whole, with forward-facing directionality in penile skin helping keep the foreskin forward until it needs to retract. In addition, directionality is an example of the efficiency of anatomical structures, which often serve more than one purpose, because, after the penis has entered the vagina, the frictional directionality of penile skin very probably helps to stretch and activate the ridged band on each thrusting stroke.

The investigators have analyzed the reliability of survey results. We are encouraged by the high level of consistency between findings in the preliminary surveys and in the web surveys. The web results are also internally consistent: Large majorities agree with both the over-all premise of the website and with specific, measurable reflexes.

The authors had cleaned the initial data to exclude so far as possible bogus or off-the-subject responses. It was fortunate for this purpose that so many respondents provided comments, which enabled us to exclude six surveys that were not from intact males.

Also, questions in the basic survey were structured to reduce bias occasioned by the normal human tendency to respond "yes" rather than "no." To support the basic premise, two of the six questions needed a "no" answer, including the key question: "Do you find the glans plays a more important role (in sexual intercourse) than the foreskin?"

We had been especially concerned about response bias occasioned by diametrically opposed viewpoints from potential respondents on the subject of infant circumcision. Before launching the website, we wondered if some circumcision enthusiasts might seek to bias the survey with faked negative responses. This clearly did not happen.

At the opposite end of the spectrum, we were concerned that some anti-circumcision activists might, in effect, stuff the ballot box. The tremendous diversity in comments received, the range of small individual differences in responses to each question, and the steady pace of responses over many months all argue against this hypothesis. Also, as shown in Table 3, an appreciable number of respondents had clearly imbibed pro-circumcision rhetoric, which is still endemic in the United States, so that responses expressing doubts about the foreskin partially balanced those from people opposed to circumcision. Concerns expressed about the foreskin covered a wide range, from extreme ("Could you tell me how to circumcise myself?" to virtually subconscious ("I plan to keep it [my foreskin] unless some medical reason should arise that would need be to cause its removal.").

We briefly examined the record of website hits to see which parts of the site get the most attention and to examine whether visitors are coming from sites that would predispose them toward response bias. There are over 1000 hits on a typical day representing hundreds of site visitors. Not surprisingly, many looked only at the pictures and saw neither the survey nor the sections about anatomy and function. However, with picture visits excluded, there appeared to be steady interest in the several other parts of the site as well.

Many visitors arrive from www.cirp.org, which has won many awards for web excellence and, in the authors' view, fairly represents the subjects that it addresses. That it does not accord equal weight to arguments for and against circumcision seems to us to reflect reality rather than bias.

Visitors also find the site through search engines like Google, which has ranked it high for the key word "prepuce." Search engines that pick up words like "prepuce," "foreskin," "glans," or "penis" are close to value-neutral.

In total, we have undertaken multiple steps to examine and minimize response bias. We believe our results are credible.

5.   SUMMARY AND CONCLUSION

Repeated, independent studies have confirmed that the human foreskin contains large concentrations of specialized sensory end-organs, which by 1996 were definitively placed in a ridged band that radiates from the frenulum. The present study commenced with preliminary tests that strongly implied an important role for the ridged band in male sexual reflexes. Preliminary tests also revealed that some circumcised males may have lost these reflexes. The authors therefore created an Internet site that describes how the ridged band appears to participate in sexual reflexes and that asks intact adult males to confirm or deny the sexual importance of the foreskin and its ridged band. Responses have affirmed both the over-all concept and each reflex element within it.

The web survey established that researchers can learn much about penile reflexes simply by asking respondents to record the presence or absence of easily observed physical changes, specifically, erection, contraction of the bulbocavernosal muscle, firming of penile skin, or change in the skin's frictional resistance, in response to simple, well-defined stimuli. The stimulation of stretch receptors in the ridged band is clearly the nexus of these reflexes. This is a somewhat surprising finding, because other types of sexual stimulus to the penis are more frequently cited, such as light touch, deep pressure, or, simply, erotic thoughts, and much more attention has been placed on the glans than on the ridged band even though both are clearly important.

In the course of the study, the investigators have described for the first time the forward-facing directionality of penile skin during erection and its tendency to firm and tighten. We also received strong support for the idea that the ridged band is even more important to sexual pleasure than the glans. An incidental finding, widely overlooked by both friends and enemies of the foreskin, is that, during erection, the foreskin typically covers more than half the glans.

We very much appreciate the open-mindedness of survey participants in learning to test unfamiliar concepts. Survey confirmation of the findings is especially significant because the concepts were completely new to the vast majority of respondents.

An important outcome of the study is the creation of a pool of articulate and foreskin-literate subjects, who have expressed their willingness to participate in further studies. The difficulty that many participants initially experienced with the questions is itself an important finding: Studies that do not provide extensive education for participants are likely to fail.

Our research about the foreskin has now extended over many years. We intend to continue investigating its role, focusing next on why the penis has related but separate sensory areas in both the glans and the foreskin.

However, evidence already in place provides compelling support for the sexual importance of the foreskin. We therefore encourage persons who counsel parents about childbirth issues to provide clear and thorough information on the sexual importance of this often-sacrificed tissue.

ACKNOWLEDGMENTS

The authors wish to acknowledge with great appreciation the wise counsel and vital computer assistance of Dennis C. Harrison, without whom this study could not have been accomplished. We also owe special thanks to Geoffrey T. Falk and to all our patient and thoughtful survey participants.

Table 2. Survey Results for Intact Adult Males

	Yes	No	Unsure	Total
Does the information on this website generally agree with your experience as an intact adult male?	181 91%	7 4%	11 6%	199 100%*
More specifically, are the descriptions of the anatomy of the foreskin and its 'ridged band' reasonably accurate, in your opinion?	181 91%	4 2%	14 7%	199 100%
If so, do you think the ridged band plays an important role in sexual intercourse?	159 80%	13 7%	26 13%	198** 100%
In your opinion, is the sexual role of the foreskin similar to that outlined on this website?	175 88%	10 5%	14 7%	199 100%
Do you find the glans plays a more important role (in sexual intercourse) than the foreskin?	53 27%	93 47%	52 26%	198** 100%
Does this site, in your opinion exaggerate the importance of the foreskin as sexual tissue?	25 13%	152 76%	22 11%	199 100%

*Does not add because of rounding

**One non-respondent

Table 3. Comments from survey respondents

Analytical/descriptive

"On the underside of my penis, where the ridged band actually joins the glans, the band is definitely more sensitive than the glans. But, on the upper side, they are about equally sensitive….My glamorous assistant would like to add that she finds a foreskin better, gives a much more pleasurable sensation and is more comfortable."

"The foreskin also provides a thin insulating layer between the penis and the vaginal orifice if left partially retracted prior to entry. . . This provides adequate protection and more pleasure for the partner of the intact male as well as greater pleasure for the intact male."

"I think the foreskin and the glans work together….One is not necessarily more important than the other, however, I could not live without either."

"[W]hen I develop an erection the sensations of the foreskin folding back across my penis head is very stimulating and gives me a lot of pleasure."

"During covert operations….I was caught and subject to questioning . . . , which included interrogators extinguishing cigarettes on my body. The application of lit cigarette ends to my glans was not anywhere near as painful as to other parts of my body, and the resultant scar tissue is less marked than elsewhere, just a darker skin."

"[W]hen I used to masturbate with the frenum intact my glans would pulsate with mini throbs of pleasure. Since I severed my cord this no longer occurs in my glans."

"One of the things I am aware of, as an intact man, is that sexual sensation in the penis is a combination of sensations in different parts."

"[W]hen [the foreskin is] retracted hard back to the base and held there, I can orgasm without the need to stimulate myself." (from a response to the follow-up survey)

Concerned or naive about the foreskin

"I do feel some foreskins are so long it must be at the very least a problem with hygiene. I have to say that I am neither pro or anti circumcision per se."

"[W]hen I get an erection, the foreskin does not retract….But I was wondering if there are any medical problems this could cause, infection or something along those lines."

"I have a tendency of ejaculating early in the intercourse....I wonder if going thru circumcision would decrease this sensitivity and give me improved control over ejaculation."

"When you get an erection is the foreskin supposed to retract fully? And if so, why doesn't mine?"

"My foreskin does not roll back at all when I am erected. Does this mean I am sexually insufficient?"

"I'm not circumcised. I always worried that at birth I was too weak to have it done."

"The foreskin does put you at odds growing up because every other boy is circumcised. A little rough in the locker room but just knowing my stimulation will far exceed their feelings will make the ridicule worth it."

"Had I chanced upon this article three decades earlier I would have felt luckier."

"I'm still debating the merits of a possible adult circumcision, but don't want to make it harder to reach a peak."

"For years, I thought that the corona and frenum were key, not the inner foreskin and ridged bands."

Positive or negative feelings about site and/or foreskin

"Good work. Seems long overdue that the male prepuce begins to be understood and — particularly for Americans — valued as the protective, functional, erogenous anatomy it is."

"Glad I've still got it!"

"I'm uncut, and I love my skin. I won't lose it."

"I'm glad I still have it."

"Was uncirc'd until my early 20s and now after 10 years feel it was the best decision I have ever made."

"I love my foreskin very much, very thankful my parents did not have me circumcised."

"Intact with no regrets."

"To me the foreskin is a very important part of sex, including masturbation."

"Can't this site be made mandatory for all new parents of baby boys?"

"I am glad that I am intact. All of my lovers have the same opinion."

Table 4. Results of follow-up survey

	Yes	No	Unsure	Total
Does stretching the foreskin and its ridged band cause erection?	49 67%	16 22%	8 11%	73 100
When you tightly stretch the foreskin and its ridged band during an erection, do you find more resistance when a finger moves firmly from the tip of the foreskin to the base of the penis, than if the finger moves in the opposite direction?	44 60%	15 20%	15 20%	74 100%
With the foreskin *forward*: Is the skin of the penis tighter and firmer when your penis is fully erect than it was when your penis was completely "soft?"	58 78%	15 20%	1 1%	74 100%
Same as previous question but with the foreskin pulled *back* to expose the glans	38 52%	28 38%	7 10%	73 100%
When you become fully erect, does your foreskin still cover more than half of the head of your penis?	57 78%	16 22%	0 0%	73 100%
Has the Ridged Band Website improved your sex life?	28 38%	14 19	31 43%	73 100%
Would you like to be included in another Internet survey about the foreskin at some later date?	74 99%	1 1%	0 0%	75 100%
Do you live in the United States	36 49%	38 51%	0 0%	74 100%

First iteration of question testing possible foreskin-bulbocavernosal reflex:

	Yes	No	Unsure	Total
With the foreskin retracted, does sharp retraction and relaxation of the "ridged band" cause sharp contraction and relaxation of the bulbocavernosal muscle? (This is the muscle that terminates urination; it is located just behind the scrotum.)	22 30%	25 34%	27 37%	74 100%*

Second iteration of question testing possible foreskin-bulbocavernosal reflex:

	Yes	No	Unsure	Total
With the penis erect and the foreskin properly retracted, does sharp further stretching of the foreskin (by hand) towards the base of the penis cause you to detect any change in the muscle just behind the scrotum?	27	10	8	45
	60%	22%	18%	100%

*Does not add because of rounding.

REFERENCES

1. Taylor JR, Lockwood AP, Taylor AJ. The prepuce: specialized mucosa of the penis and its loss to circumcision. Br J Urol 1996;77:291-5.
2. Winkelmann RK. The erogenous zones: their nerve supply and its significance. Proceedings of the Staff Meetings of the Mayo Clinic 1959;34:39-47. [here, p. 40].
3. Winkelmann RK. The erogenous zones: their nerve supply and its significance. Proceedings of the Staff Meetings of the Mayo Clinic 1959;34:39-47. [here, p. 41].
4. Winkelmann RK. The erogenous zones: their nerve supply and its significance. Proceedings of the Staff Meetings of the Mayo Clinic 1959;34:39-47. [here, p. 42].
5. Winkelmann RK. The cutaneous innervation of human newborn prepuce. J Invest Dermat 1956;26:53-67. [here, p. 64].
6. Winkelmann RK. The cutaneous innervation of human newborn prepuce. J Invest Dermat 1956;26:53-67. [here, p. 53.]
7. Winkelmann RK. The cutaneous innervation of human newborn prepuce. J Invest Dermat 1956;26:53-67. [here, p. 54.]
8. American Academy of Pediatrics. Circumcision policy statement. Pediatrics 1999;103:686-93. [here, p. 687.]
9. Taylor JR, Lockwood AP, Taylor AJ. The prepuce: specialized mucosa of the penis and its loss to circumcision. Br J Urol 1996;77:291-5. [here, p. 291].
10. Circumcision. Harv Men's Health Watch October 2001. URL: http://www.health.harvard.edu/newsletters. [retracted]. The same article is in print: Price C. Circumcision. Harv Mens Health Watch 2001 Oct;6(3):6-8.
11. Cold CJ, Hubbard GE, Tarara RP, Stribling LJV. Comparative anatomy of the specialized sensory receptors of the primate penis and prepuce: humans, baboons, rhesus monkeys, and marmosets. In: Conference Proceedings of The Apes: Challenges for the 21st Century; 2000 May 10-13; Brookfield, Illinois, USA:Chicago Zoological Society; 2001.URL: http://www.brookfieldzoo.org/0.asp?nSection=14&PageID=196&nLinkID=31
12. Cold CJ, McGrath KA. Anatomy and histology of the penile and clitoral prepuce in primates. In: Denniston GC, Milos MF, editors. Male and female circumcision. New York: Kluwer Academic/Plenum Publishing; 1999. pp. 19-29.
13. Cold CJ, Taylor JR. The prepuce. Br J Urol 1999:83 Suppl 1:34-44. [here, p. 40.]

Chapter 4

CIRCUMCISION AND SEXUAL PLEASURE

George C Denniston MD, MPH
Clinical Assistant Professor, Department of Family Medicine, University of Washington, Seattle, Washington

Abstract: Thirty—eight (38) men who had experienced sexual intercourse *before* they were circumcised are members of an elite group who have experienced the qualitative differences in sexual pleasure between the circumcised and the intact state. This study asked these men for the advantages, and the disadvantages of circumcision. Twenty—four (24) men *volunteered* "decreased sensitivity" as a disadvantage. Direct quotations describe their feelings about the loss of half of the skin from their normal penis.

Key words: Circumcision, phimosis, paraphimosis, ridged band, pain, ejaculation

1.   INTRODUCTION

This study was designed to gain insight into the relationship between circumcision and sexual pleasure.

2.   METHODS

A request for volunteers for a study was sent out via a notice in the NOCIRC Annual Report (National Organization of Circumcision Information Resource Centers, San Anselmo, CA) for men who were circumcised after age eighteen. No additional information was given. Seventy-one (71) men volunteered, over a five-month period, to participate in the study. Each was sent a two-page questionnaire and a return envelope. Fifty-two (52) men returned the study.

Flesh and Blood, Edited by Denniston et al.
Kluwer Academic/Plenum Publishers, New York 2004

Without divulging the precise nature of the study, we specifically asked about age at first intercourse, as well as birth date and age at circumcision. Final admission to the study required that the men be sexually active for a minimum of two years before their circumcision. Thirty-eight (38) men were qualified by the above criterion to enter the study. Because these men volunteered, they do not constitute a representative sample, so they do not necessarily describe the situation in any larger group of men, such as all American men. We present here 38 case reports.

3.   RESULTS

Thirty-eight (38) men, who had experienced sexual intercourse before and after circumcision, were included in the study. The age at circumcision among the 38 sexually active males was 18 to 54 years. Fifty-three percent (53%) were between 20 and 29 years of age. (Figure 1)

The reasons for having an adult circumcision fell into three categories.

One group requested circumcision because, for years, they felt they did not "measure up." They had been ridiculed for being intact and had been given no help in recognizing they were normal, so they requested circumcision.

A second group was circumcised during military duty. They entered the Armed Services and, one way or another, ended up circumcised.

The third group had medical, or what they thought was a medical reasons for having it done. Whether or not circumcision is used to "treat" a given condition depends largely on whether or not the doctor intends to preserve an intact penis. None of the doctors seen by the individuals in this study recognized the importance of an intact and were of that persuasion.

After the men in this study had their circumcision performed, many said they were satisfied with the results, and many said they regretted their decision. The proportion of those who regretted their circumcision varied with the reason for having the circumcision performed. The men who regretted it least were the ones who requested the circumcision. But, even when they requested it, fully fifty percent (50%) of those who requested circumcision regretted it in the time frame of this study. (Table 1)

Satisfaction with the circumcision was strongly correlated with whether or not sexual intercourse was perceived as better after circumcision. (Table 2) Thirteen men felt that intercourse was better and would have the circumcision again. Twenty-two men felt that intercourse was worse and would not have the circumcision again.

Of the thirteen (13) men who would have the circumcision again, and for whom sexual intercourse was better, ten (10) men came from the group that requested it. [Two men had more than one reason.] (Table 3)

The men were asked "What are the advantages of the procedure for you?" And "What are the disadvantages for you?" Each man gave one or more answers.

3.1   Advantages

A. Some of these men stated there were no advantages (11). The number in parentheses is the number of men who volunteered that response.

B. Others wrote that they felt more comfortable. These include feeling better in the locker room (5), appearance (12), comfort (2), women prefer it (4), and a "greater sense of belonging" (1).

C. Another group of advantages falls under the heading of "improved health." These include cleanliness (16), easier to urinate (5), "relief of slight paraphimosis (constriction following retraction)" (1), other alleged medical reasons(2) ("phimosis" – a normal constriction of the opening in the prepuce, which may persist, but is now known to be harmless).

D. Other advantages noted are improved sexual relations, including intercourse is better (4), more intensity during intercourse (4), easier penetration (2), delayed ejaculation (2), partner willing to give increased oral stimulation (1), "glans not so sensitive" (1), and persistent sexual feelings due to skin tightness (1).

3.2   Disadvantages

A. One man stated there were no disadvantages (1).

B. Some men stated that masturbation was less enjoyable (8) and more difficult (4), foreplay was less enjoyable (1), foreplay for the partner was less enjoyable (1), penetration was more difficult (3), and erection was more difficult to obtain and retain (2). There was decreased sensitivity of the glans (19), decreased sensitivity during intercourse (4), decreased intensity of orgasm (2), intercourse was less enjoyable (4),oral sex was not as pleasurable (1), intercourse took too long (6), and there were fewer orgasms (1). Some stated they were aware of the loss of sensitive tissue (6), and "complete loss of my normal sexual ability" (1). Some experienced less comfort (8). One man described it as "loss of ecstasy" (1),one felt "naked" (1), and one "felt incomplete" (1).

The most striking result is that 24 men, when asked the open-ended question, "What are the disadvantages of circumcision?" replied, *in their own handwriting*, "decreased sensitivity." This reply was not obtained by checking options on a multiple-choice question.

The men made comments about whether or not circumcision harmed them.

3.3 Direct Quotations

#2 "Less pleasurable than before. It was better for partner – the extra skin moving around. I had it cut off to look like others. I felt very comfortable with my circumcision. Now I'm stretching foreskin back – head again covered – sensitivity is returning. Sexual relations have been better in the last six months than they have been in years." (This man had his circumcision 33 years ago. This case attests to the unacceptable loss of sensitivity with age, which demands further study.)

#3 "I have always wanted it done, from the first time I was old enough to be aware of the difference."

#8 "The skin removed was very sensitive, particularly at the tip and underneath. An orgasm was a combination of greater sensitivity over a larger area. Less control, the skin covering the head reduces level of arousal and extends duration before ejaculation."

#9 "The procedure always leaves the person less sensitive and dry. Being dry, penetration requires lubricant. The foreskin sensitivity greatly enhances intercourse and the 'feeling' prior to my circumcision was 100 times better. I have lost sensitivity to the extent that it is difficult to tell if penetration has occurred. Prior to circumcision, every movement was ecstasy – now intercourse is mental rather than physical."

#11 "My foreskin gathered behind the glans and rubbed the inside of the vagina and the clitoris like a French tickler. My orgasms are not as pleasurable now. With a foreskin, I was capable of many erections and ejaculations because my glans was more sensitive."

#13 "I believe I would have benefited from infant circumcision, but I can understand why an increasing number of people are opposed to it."

#14 "I think it was the worst mistake I ever made."

#17 "A lot of what were very good feelings are gone. I wish I still had a foreskin."

#18 "My foreskin used to guide me right in. It would catch on my partner's outer lips and then roll back as my head came out. The head is much less sensitive. Sometimes I won't ejaculate at all, even after 45 minutes of thrusting." [Prolonged thrusting of a calloused glans is obviously a major cause of dyspareunia (painful intercourse) for the female partner.]

#19 "No feeling whatsoever in the head. All sensation is in what used to be the inside of the foreskin, and most of that was removed. Ejaculation has been turned into a goal, rather than a pleasure. I feel like the only authorities on circumcision are those of us who have experienced both conditions."

#20 "I always thought my foreskin looked ugly. I had it done because of personal hygiene and the aesthetic of it."

#21 "My penile skin now very tight, flaccid and erect, causing a bend in my penis when erect. I have full loss of sensitivity in the glans. Still, on occasions, I have some discomfort with penile and scrotal skin tightness, mainly erect, when the skin is very tight. Ejaculation is now weak. slow, and takes a long while to arrive and finish."

#22 "When a man loses the central nervous system of his penis, he loses the control of his orgasm, and the control of his penis. Sex becomes a workout, not love."

#24 "I have been most happy that I made the decision, but sorry it was not made during infancy."

#27 "My wife wanted it done. She didn't like the way I looked and was afraid of getting cancer because I was not circumcised. She thought it would be cleaner also. Circumcision has reduced my sexual pleasure and sensation to the degree that I wish I had never had it done."

#29 "Everything available to read back then (1967) indicated it would make your sex life much better and make you a better lover."

#30 "I only reach orgasm one time. Before I reached orgasm 2 to 3 times."

#31 "???"

#32 "It just doesn't feel as good as it did with the foreskin intact."

#33 "I firmly believe that if men who were circumcised as infants, were ever able to compare sensation with a foreskin and without, they would storm the hospitals before they would allow such mutilation to be performed on their own boys."

#35 "Gentle strokes and sensitive nerve endings are more important than violent thrusts and a long ride."

#36 My brother had had his foreskin stretched successfully. At age 18, I was in the office of a country doctor – no anesthesia. After a quick exam, I was strapped to the exam table. Forceps were clamped to the end of my foreskin. It was pulled forward as far as possible. I thought he was just stretching it. I closed my eyes. I then felt the worst pain of my life. Opening my eyes, I saw my foreskin in his forceps and blood all over my penis and elsewhere."

#36 We have a 32—year—old uncircumcised [intact] son and he has thanked us for sparing him the cut."

#37 "Loss of sensitivity. Loss of something unique that cannot be replaced."

4.   DISCUSSION

Men who have been circumcised after they have experienced sexual intercourse while intact are the only heterosexual men in the world with experience of the qualitative differences between the intact and the circumcised state as it relates to sexual pleasure.

Several of these men provide an accurate description of what happens when a penis loses one-half of its normal skin, the half that contains the major organ of sexual pleasure, the ridged band. After circumcision, the penile skin is no longer loose and mobile during erection, as it is on all normal mammals (#21). The glans becomes calloused and loses its sensitivity. The extensive network of sensitive nerve endings in the foreskin, especially the ridged band, has been amputated)(#9). Ejaculation is weak and slow (#21). Once multi-orgasmic, now a man can have only one orgasm (#30). There is a "loss of something unique that cannot be replaced"(#37). Parents contemplating circumcision for their son must be informed of all these adverse effects.

An inherent bias exists in virtually all of the responses. Each of these men was circumcised in a society where the medical priesthood had ordained that circumcision was a good thing. One subject (#29) put it succinctly: "Everything available to read back then (1967) indicated it would make your sex life much better and make you a better lover." So many men who reported benefits received psychological benefits, rather than physical ones.

Most of the medical information they received was incorrect. One striking example of this was the man (#27) whose wife wanted him to be circumcised to prevent her from getting cancer. The scientific world dismissed circumcision as an alleged cause of cervical cancer more than twenty years ago.

Men who stated that circumcision had advantages were influenced by propaganda and may have been overstating the benefits. Those who stated that circumcision had disadvantages were speaking against the dominant paradigm. Going against the prevailing myths took courage and meant that they were much more likely to be reporting the results accurately. In fact, they may well have been understating the harm done to them. With this bias in mind, we may now look at the numerical results once again.

Eleven (11) men said there were no advantages to circumcision.

The advantages presented under B in Results, "More comfortable," constitute important psychological reasons to be circumcised in a world where most men are circumcised, but disappear in a world where the majority is intact.

The advantages mentioned under C in Results, alleging improved health, are easily handled without resorting to circumcision. For cleanliness, intact males easily retract the loose, mobile foreskin while bathing, and have no more difficulty cleaning their penis than a circumcised male. If this is difficult (in rare instances of persistent phimosis or paraphimosis), gentle stretching cures the problem.

The advantages of improved sexual relations, noted under D, may sometimes be achieved by circumcision in adulthood for those men who wish it, with fully informed consent. Of course, this study documents that circumcision often does not achieve improvement in sexual relations. The rate of regret is already 50%, and it can easily go higher as the men get older.

4.1   Functions of the Foreskin

The foreskin has a number of functions throughout the life of a man. It is important that everyone understand these functions.

Before birth, the foreskin covers the glans and is completely attached to the glans. When a male is born, the foreskin is still attached to the glans (in 96% of boys). This skin protects the glans, just as the eyelid protects the eye, and as all skin protects body organs. Urine is released and, if the foreskin is left alone – never retracted until it separates naturally, difficulties are rarely encountered.

Throughout infancy and childhood in the intact male, the foreskin continues to protect the sensitive glans. After the foreskin finally separates from the glans by a fascinating natural process,[1-2] the space under the foreskin can be made to disappear simply by retracting the loose foreskin. The penis then appears to look just like the circumcised penis.

As the boy matures into a man, the foreskin plays an even more vital role. With erection of the penis, an function necessary for the continuation of the species, the shaft of the penis increases in length by at least 50%. Where does the additional skin come from to cover the longer shaft? It is the foreskin that provides the covering for this enlarged organ. The intact male often has enough foreskin to cover part of the glans. Maximum sensitivity is achieved when the inside of the foreskin, containing tiny sensitive ridges, rubs over the rim, or corona of the glans.

Another function of the foreskin is to provide exquisite sensations that are intimately linked to the reproductive process. New studies of the inner portion of the intact foreskin show it to be more complex, and to have more nerve endings, than the surface of the glans. A series of tiny ridges, the ridged bands, have been identified as the organ of sensitivity.[3] The foreskin is not an appendage. It is the skin of the penis with functions of its own.

4.2   Circumcision Pain

Until recently, many doctors denied that the infant experienced pain during circumcision. Mothers who have heard the screams affirm their child's pain, and experienced pediatricians acknowledge that the screams during a foreskin amputation are qualitatively different from other crying. With the publication of Anand and Hickey's classic paper in the *New England Journal of Medicine* in 1987, doctors can no longer reasonably deny that an infant experiences pain.[4] Anesthesia for the circumcision does nothing for the succeeding weeks of pain and discomfort in this sensitive area.

4.3   Circumcision Contraindicated

Removing the foreskin of a newborn infant or young boy is almost always unnecessary. In rare instances, if the infant cannot urinate, simple stretching can enlarge the opening of the foreskin. Otherwise, it is to be left alone, to separate gradually from the glans, and to develop normally. Two hundred and fifty million (250,000,000) European men, with access to excellent medical care, remain intact all of their life, and rarely permit anyone to remove their foreskin. Many of them cannot believe that we practice routine circumcision in America.

The testimony of the men in this study about decreased sexual sensitivity, coupled with an understanding of the functions of the foreskin, the recent findings regarding the infant's capacity for experiencing pain, and the fact that most of the men in the world live happily with their foreskin should be enough to ensure that all male infants are permitted to retain their natural body parts until they come of age. As adults, they can decide for themselves whether or not to have their foreskin removed. With the available evidence that men who are circumcised are deprived of much of their sexual sensitivity, no physician should want to take the risk of significantly harming a patient under his or her care.

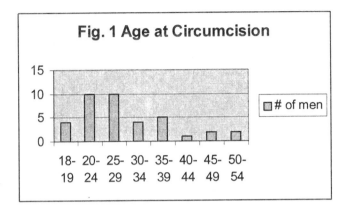

Figure 1. Age at Circumcision

Table 1. "Would you have it again?"

Reason for having circumcision performed	Yes	No
Requested circumcision	8	8 (50%)
Military	1	4 (80%)
"Medical"	6	11 (64%)

Table 2. "Would you have it again?"

After circumcision, is intercourse...	Yes	No
better	13	0
worse	0	22
no change	2	1

Table 3. "Yes, I would have it again and sexual intercourse is better."

Reason for having circumcision performed.	
Requested circumcision	10
Military	1
"Medical"	4

REFERENCES

1. Hunter RH. Notes on the development of the prepuce. J. Anat 1935; 70:68-75
2. Gairdner D. The Fate of the Foreskin. BMJ 1949; 2:1433-7.
3. Taylor JR, Lockwood AP, Taylor AJ. The prepuce: specialized mucosa of the penis and its loss to circumcision. Br J Urol 1996; 77:291-5
4. Anand KJS, Hickey PR. Pain and its effects in the human neonate and fetus. NEJM 1987; 317:1321-9

Chapter 5

CONSERVATIVE TREATMENT OF PRIMARY PREPUTIAL STENOSIS IN ADOLESCENTS

Michel Beaugé, MD
Vice Chairman of the National Union of Sexologists, and the Secretary General of the Group of Western France Sexologists for Advanced Training. Quimper, France.

Abstract: This paper describes a conservative method of widening the preputial ring in cases of preputial stenosis in adolescent males. Prescription of kinestherapy is effective in widening the preputial ring. Resolution of the preputial stenosis can be achieved in a few weeks. In the absence of cutaneous abnormalities, manual remodeling of the foreskin of the foreskin allows the avoidance of surgical intervention and spares the patient from all of the unavoidable problems and disadvantages that result when surgery is performed.

Key words: phimosis, preputial stenosis, circumcision

1.   INTRODUCTION

Being in charge of the routine examination of college freshmen as part of the preventive medicine program of the university in Quimper for more than ten years, I diagnose a significant amount of preputial stenosis in adults.

Among this male population, aged eighteen to twenty-two, we have observed that nearly ten percent have various degrees of tightness of the foreskin, ranging from total inability to expose the glans to a simple ring that gets stuck in the sulcus. In this report, the word phimosis, indicating preputial stenosis, means that the diameter of the inferior preputial ring is smaller than the diameter of the corona of the erect glans.

From the interviews, it appears that the great majority of these males are virgins and that, among those who have had sexual experience, many have failed because of difficulty in penetration, pain, and loss of erection; except perhaps in cases of the greatest stenosis who were successful in penile penetration with the glans covered. The remainder is at considerable risk of paraphimosis should they persevere in intercourse. The possibility of paraphimosis, as well as the difficulties in carrying out successful intercourse, often make it prudent to intervene medically.

2.   TREATMENT

The conventional treatment of phimosis is surgical: Circumcision, which removes the foreskin, or simple plastic surgery, which preserves the fold of skin but widens the orifice. For a number of reasons, I have come to reject these radical therapeutic procedures because surgical intervention is traumatic, brutal, irreversible, and bloody, and because it requires anesthesia.

The two latter features give rise to possible complications similar to any other form of surgery. Plastic surgery may fail due to scar formation. Circumcision is especially egregious because it reduces the mobility of the penile skin by amputating a large part of it. Furthermore, circumcision is psychologically stressful because it cuts the sexual organ, which is highly symbolic for a male at the dawn of his sexual life; it creates a mutilation; it causes the penis to look different from that of friends at an age when the young man has scarcely acquired knowledge of normality; it causes brutal exposure of the mucous membrane by the excision of the protection of the glans; it interferes with the pattern of masturbation — a consequence that may be seriously traumatic. Finally, circumcision is expensive and requires hospitalization.

Remodeling of the foreskin should be considered because it is painless, gradual, unobtrusive, free of cost, non-traumatic, and trouble-free. Additional and more significant advantages of remodeling are that it preserves the foreskin and its important and irreplaceable functions, allows the preservation of patterns of masturbation, and avoids the pain of the exposed glans. It is logical to consider surgery only for those rare cases where remodeling fails to achieve the desired ends.

3.   REFLECTIONS

The study of observed cases reveals that adolescent or young adult subjects suffering from preputial stenosis have habits of masturbation different from others.

Conventionally, the pursuit of solitary pleasure is done with the dominant hand closed over the penis making alternate back and forth movement over the shaft, the hand going down towards the pubis, uncovering the glans, which the index finger or thumb may now and then lightly stroke, reproducing the sensation of intercourse.

This exercise results in moving the penile skin in the same way it occurs in vaginal intercourse and, therefore, serves as a valuable preparation for adult sexual relations. We shall see later that this training is not only mechanical, but also contributes to the psychological development of the individual.

I have established a classification of the methods of masturbation reported by patients with a stenotic prepuce.

1. Some boys never masturbate. We may doubt their assertions, but the preputial orifice's resistance to retraction suggests that their statements are truthful. In these cases, ejaculation takes place during sleep (nocturnal emissions) and, more rarely, spontaneously while awake, prompted by stimulating events among those subjects who attach guilt to contact with the penis.

2. Others stroke the glans through the medium of the foreskin in the usual way, but attempt to pull the skin towards the tip of the penis instead of pulling it back toward the pubis. Among these boys, we find the persistence of a long tubular foreskin such as is seen in infants.

3. In some cases, the boy rolls the penis between two palms or between one hand and another surface such as the abdomen, the thigh, a table, the edge of a chair (in particular the toilet). It is usual in these cases for the raphe on the underside of the penis not to be in the midline but more or less displaced to one side or even spiral; the preputial orifice is often displaced.

4. Mechanical stimulation without use of the hands is found most frequently, among those suffering from guilt resulting from the consequences of anti-sex indoctrination. In general, the boy, flat on his face on his bed, labors as if for intercourse with the help of his pelvic musculature, and rubs his penis against the mattress, the bolster or a pillow, often through a cover in which — sign of the times — he has placed a disposable paper tissue to avoid stains that would betray his activity to his mother.

5. Interfemoral stimulation is found, facilitated by a penis curved downward, unless it is this activity that determines the anatomical anomaly. This technique has an advantage in that it can be carried out in

company, much as some females have orgasms by squeezing their thighs, while climbing a rope, or while riding a bicycle.

6. Instrumental masturbation can be achieved by mechanical vibrator or by showering, but it has never been demonstrated in the population under consideration and therefore must be rare or of occasional practice.

7. For the record, auto-fellatio, when mobility allows it.

4.   ROLES OF MASTURBATION

Following this analysis, we may consider that masturbation serves many useful and healthful purposes.

1. Masturbation serves to evacuate the accumulated store of semen produced by a pubescent boy. The tension felt by men after a certain time following the last ejaculation is well known.

2. Masturbation is enjoyable. A boy who has discovered that he can elicit pleasure through the mechanical stimulation of his penis recreates the conditions of this pleasure, and this effort is rewarded by orgasm,

3. Masturbation allows the subject to learn how to obtain orgasmic sensations and also how to recognize the erogenous stimuli that create them. Masturbation enables him to perceive the beginning of ejaculation and, therefore, to find ways to prevent it, if desirable. No doubt, the regular practice of this activity forms the basis for the avoidance of premature ejaculation. Variations are possible on the theme of sexual pleasure, and masturbation affords an opportunity to explore the field of eroticism.

4. Masturbation has a role in preparing the penis for its future purpose and serves to overcome organic obstacles to penetration. The basis of the therapeutic procedure I will describe is based on an understanding of how handling the penis effects the development of the foreskin and the elimination of preputial stenosis.

Indeed, it is apparent that the number of males with preputial stenosis decreases with age. Inability to retract the foreskin is normal in infants, common among young boys, but only persists in about ten percent of the subjects at the end of adolescence.

5. Finally, masturbation contributes to fantasy life and helps the subject to structure himself mentally for his future life.

5. THERAPEUTIC PROCEDURE

When consulted by a man with a stenotic prepuce, it is important first to make an analysis of the patient's method of masturbation. It is necessary to explain to him the useful functions of masturbation during adolescence, as described in the five preceding points.

The discussion has the advantage of dispelling misinformation and feelings of guilt, if present. Unfortunately, some males wrongly believe that they are not supposed to touch the penis. Some believe it does not belong to them, or they feel that the penis is taboo. Some males may be afraid to uncover the glans because they imagine that it might fall off. Sadly, some males, as children, are instructed that they are not supposed to experience sexual pleasure.

The discussion may also be helpful in other areas. For instance, some males were never shown how to clean their penis. Some males have been traumatized by clumsy and painful efforts by doctors or parents to examine the child's penis, a regrettable occurrence that may have negative consequences for the future psychosexual development of the male.

Next, it is advisable to instruct the patient about the masturbatory technique that seems to be most useful, such as gently pulling back the foreskin and attempting to expose just the tip of the glans. It is only rarely possible for a boy who has developed a method that leads to orgasm to replace it initially by another. Generally, the new method fails to give pleasure and may even tend to impair the quality of the erection. This could explain why boys fail in their first attempts at sexual intercourse; a man who has become accustomed to rotational movements on his penis for several years will be quite unable to use this technique in the vagina. Therefore, I advise alternating a few pleasurable manipulations known to be stimulating with the remodeling manipulations. It is of course essential that the preputial opening be stretched round the circumference of the fully erect glans. This technique meets the requirements of the kinestherapy of soft tissues, gradual stretching the orifice to attain a permanently wider circumference. In some cases, I have recommended instrumental dilatation with the use of a dilator in patients who agree to this procedure, or I have advised the introduction of two fingers into the opening of the foreskin to dilate it.

Perhaps it is logical to draw a parallel between the preputial ring of the boy and the hymen of the girl. In both cases, there is a mucocutaneous stricture that obstructs intercourse while still allowing the passage of urine and, in the case of the hymen, the flow of menses. The opening of the hymen may occur through traumatic rupture during brutal penetration or by gradual and gentle dilatation when the lover is careful or shy.

Whether it be the prepuce or hymen, it is the erect glans that serves as the biologically correct dilator that models the orifice appropriately.

Using this remodeling technique, the boy can progressively expand his foreskin until the diameter is equal to that of the erect glans, allowing him subsequently to proceed to sexual intercourse without risk of paraphimosis.

During the course of this remodeling, there will come a time when the preputial orifice is sufficiently dilated to uncover the distal part of the glans but is still too narrow to go over the proximal and larger part of the glans. This is due to the conical shape of the glans. We can then imagine that a strong enough pull might succeed in sliding the ring into the sulcus, but that the reverse movement might be impossible, causing paraphimosis during masturbation. This appears to me unlikely for several reasons. First, the manipulation is done under visual control of the subject who is well able to detect the degree of tension in the foreskin, unlike the situation during sexual intercourse, particularly when it occurs for the first time;

Second, if paraphimosis nevertheless did occur in this situation, it could only be moderately tight and would be reduced immediately by the subject who is free to readjust himself at his convenience. Furthermore, in this situation, orgasm would not occur. Masturbation would be stopped at once and the secondary increase in volume and firmness of the glans would not take place. In coital paraphimosis, the foreskin enters the sulcus during intercourse and then orgasm causes further increase in volume and firmness of the glans making reduction more difficult. Finally, the boy's embarrassment at manipulating himself in the presence of his partner to reduce the foreskin, explains the delay during which edema collects and the condition becomes established.

6.   RESULTS

I have recommended this treatment for thirty to forty boys annually and therefore have observed several hundred cases. Follow-up in preventive medicine is not usual and many were not seen again, however, about half did return to report a satisfactory outcome. Some of them, grateful to have benefited from such a gentle and discreet treatment method, entrusted me with other problems and therefore have provided accounts of the success of the treatment over a longer period. With regard to patients from my town, a number were given the same advice and I reckon that, in fifteen years of practice, I never had to refer a single one for surgery.

In a few cases, patients agreed to be photographed with the foreskin stretched on the erect glans at the start, with a second photograph taken four weeks later. These demonstrate that retraction of the foreskin was achieved, as a rule, within this time. The outcomes occurred in the same time as that of the scar formation after surgery. These results, therefore, encourage the use of this technique.

I did not come across any failures, but this does not mean that they did not occur since such cases may have failed to return for follow-up. It should be pointed out that an attempt at conservative treatment does not prevent subsequent recourse to surgery.

7.   DISCUSSION

If we must criticize the proposed method of reducing preputial stenosis through masturbation-based remodeling technique, we must ask ourselves two questions: First, is it permissible to discuss masturbation with these boys? And second, should circumcision be rejected?

As for the propriety of masturbation, we note that masturbation is universal in humans. It occurs in all young children and is the usual form of sexual expression among Western adolescents. Gerard Mendel in *Anthropologie Differentielle* points out that "If we recall the universality of infantile masturbation during the first years and the near-universality in adolescent boys, we realize then what a role it must take."[1]

In our society, adolescence tends to be prolonged voluntarily into the third decade and masturbation continues in these young single men. Some married men make up for the difference in their and their partner's libido by taking a mistress. Men may temporarily or permanently be alone, whether willingly or unwillingly as a result of life's vicissitudes. Masturbation also forms part of the sexual relationship of couples, and a woman will masturbate her partner to avoid intercourse, which may be undesirable for various reasons. A young girl, for instance, may prefer to delay her first intercourse. She may prefer to avoid intercourse because of menstruation, vulvo-vaginal irritation, or because of a fear of pregnancy. Finally, she may prefer to masturbate her partner and avoid intercourse because of a healthy interest in the functions and mechanics of the penis.

The symbolism of masturbation is found everywhere in daily life and humor, for example, the shaken champagne bottle ejaculating foam in the hands of the winner of a motor race. Masturbation is also a well known means of obtaining or reviving an erection when mental stimulation is insufficient. Additionally, masturbation is still the primary method of "safe sex" as advised for the avoidance of HIV infection and even recommended by certain governments, e.g., Canada.

The usefulness of masturbation is also proven in other medical arenas. Masturbation is advised twice weekly as adjuvant treatment of chronic prostatitis in single men.

Our senses of sight, hearing, and smell have been developed to ensure survival by detecting predators so that we can defend ourselves against them, as well as to capture prey and obtain food. Today, in our society, these senses are extensively exploited to obtain pleasure from pictures, music, sculpture, and perfumes. Likewise, the sense of taste necessary to recognize wholesome food is exploited in cooking and even in tobacco smoking and the enjoyment of wine.

We admit that civilization allows us this leeway in the use of our sense organs. We have freed sexual and sensual pleasure from the confines of reproduction and survival of the species (who would be satisfied with intercourse three or four times in their life?). We can, therefore, allow sexuality to be expressed freely by individual choice (within the limits of the liberty of others), and free ourselves from the biblical guilt surrounding sex. Masturbation has its place within the range of sexual expression, and morality has no rational arguments to displace it.

Sigmund Freud even noted that: "I have come to believe that masturbation is the only great habit, the primitive need and that other appetites, such as the need for alcohol, morphine, tobacco, are only substitutes, the products of replacement."[2]

Contemporary western sexology emphasizes the quality of loving and spiritual relationships in the success of sexuality. This is very laudable and noble, and also frequently true, but, in fact, is neither sufficient nor indispensable. Sexual technique and the characteristics of the genital organs also play a part in successful sex. One need only analyze the factors of sexual nomadism and even prostitution to convince oneself of this.

The fact that masturbation has a role in the acquisition of sexual technique and contributes to morphological development is sufficient to justify it.

We may often be tempted to reduce masturbation to a solitary pleasure derived from mechanical stimulation of the genitals. It is not so. There is no doubt that masturbation is an antidepressant and stress reducer if it is freed from the unhealthy and damaging feelings of guilt. This sexual activity distances the individual from the worries and constraints of daily life, lulling him to sleep, whereas the pre-existing depressed state of mind would have prevented sleep. By ejaculating, the adolescent sends himself to sleep just as infants and some older children do by sucking their thumb for comfort.

Furthermore, underlying all masturbation, there is, at the psychological level, both conscious and subconscious fantasizing. Thus, the adolescent dreams and rehearses (as in repeated theatrical performances) sexual relationships that are as yet unattainable. In this sense, when he comes to his first sexual relationship, he is not entirely virgin, innocent and inexperienced.

Autoeroticism and fantasizing are described by Gerard Mendel as "productions of the same nature, that is to say, of a mnemonic, associative, and secondary nature."[3] Furthermore, "[M]asturbation is in the last resort only the means to recall, of renewing intensely the memory of the pleasure arising from the penis, as well as the whole range of sensory memories which, when stimulated, constitute fantasy."[4] Therefore, we must free our society of misplaced guilt of socio-cultural origin.

Consequently, we can conclude that masturbation is normal, natural, healthy, and perhaps even necessary. It seems permissible and prudent to advise an adolescent to direct himself towards a technique that relates to sexual intercourse.

8.   CIRCUMCISION

The glans is a precious part of the male, and, in our minds, we know that objects of value are kept in a case. Circumcision is the destruction of this case.

Circumcision is also perceived by the patient subjected to it as a partial castration. It removes part of the genitals and is therefore particularly significant on the symbolic level. Usually, the patient is ignorant, as are most doctors, about the functions of the foreskin, which means that the amount of loss and of damage is unquantified and therefore unlimited.

Circumcision is akin to amputation of the clitoral hood of the girl, which disgusts us because it is often proposed with the ulterior motive of preventing masturbation while preserving the ability to procreate. This attack on sexuality is still present in people's minds, and it should be noted that, even if the operation of the girl does not occur in France in its severest forms, it has nevertheless been justified in an insidious way with ideas such as "an honest woman must not enjoy any pleasure" and the sexual relationship between the couple is a "conjugal duty," like other chores. All practitioners in the field of sexology are familiar with the damage that such ideas continue to produce in the sexual lives of a great many female and male patients.

Mankind in general, and especially adolescents, fears genital abnormality, though primarily in terms of size rather than form or ability for sexual function. This fear is fuelled by the usual boasting on the school playground. On this sensitive ground, an amputation increases this notion of abnormality and inadequacy.

More objectively, the operation results in an aesthetic disfigurement, raising the serious risk that the patient will regard himself as disfigured.[5] A circumcised male may be disgusted by the appearance of his penis, and his partners may be disturbed by the sight of a scared shaft and permanently externalized glans. When one considers how fragile and sensitive to emotional disturbances sexual function is, one gets an idea of the alarming consequences that may result from this mutilation.

The foreskin is also an important erogenous zone.[6-7] It is one of the first such zones discovered by the infant and is the site of the erogenous trigger, particularly effective at producing an erection since the glans has only a moderate sensitivity. It seems also that stroking the foreskin is particularly good for maintaining the erect state without precipitating orgasm. An informed partner discovers these properties and knows very well how to communicate lasting sensations of high quality through the foreskin. Circumcision removes the nerve endings of this skin surface, depriving the subject of this delightful sensation. By externalizing the glans, it also results in the gradual desensitization of that structure as its delicate mucosa is overlaid with layers of sclerotic keratin. Apart from the foreskin's own sensitivity, the loss by circumcision of indirect stimulation of the glans must be taken into account, and the need to discover, with more or less difficulty, a new technique of masturbation. All of these factors contribute to the unavoidable sexual disadvantages consequent to circumcision.[8]

The foreskin can be seen as the eyelid of the glans. Its ablation denudes the mucosa of the glans and causes a dreadfully severe burning pain that the patient could well do without. The fragility and delicacy of the mucosa of the glans explain why stimulation by direct digital massage becomes painful at once. On the other hand, it is bearable and even delightful when the stimulation, instead of being direct, is carried out indirectly through the folds of the foreskin because the pressure receptors are stimulated. There are variations of pressure within the glans rather than friction or rubbing on its mucosa. The nerve endings are not tactile but sensitive to pressure. Note, too, that masturbation massages the corpus spongiosum, propelling blood towards the glans, and each wave increases the pressure there.

Dr. Gerard Zwang expresses the same ideas in rich and well-chosen words: "The child acquires...the experience of conscious sexual pleasure by practicing this delicious handling of the penis indirectly through the foreskin. The only frictional contact that the glans appreciates, savors and tolerates is that of the moist and padded vaginal (or oral) mucosa. The rough, dry friction of the hand or of the fingers would soon become unbearable if Mother Nature in her wisdom had not interposed the foreskin as a screen between the stimulating hand and the very delicate primary erogenous epithelium. The to and fro movement of the foreskin on the glans, nicely eased by the lubricating sebaceous coating, gives rise to this alternating stimulation, which is an effective method of producing orgasm."[9]

Circumcision seems to cause a rapid tensing of the frenulum (should it survive the surgery undamaged) during penetration and could contribute to premature ejaculation.

Above all, it is the loss of the reserve of skin provided by the foreskin that damages the physiology of coitus. In evolutionary terms, the primary function of the foreskin is to allow vaginal intercourse to take place under optimal conditions without friction between the mucosal surfaces of the two participants.

To illustrate this faculty, a genitally intact boy can, as a rule, move his fingers from the tip of the foreskin to the base of the penis without causing the slightest slippage on the skin. The foreskin unrolls. This skin slides on the penis. Its length and elasticity allow it to travel the entire length of the organ. There is no other part of the body where the subcutaneous tissues allow such mobility.

This explains why sexual intercourse with the intact penis can be prolonged without causing friction and therefore irritation of the surfaces in contact, i.e., the penile skin and the vaginal mucosa. The movement does not occur between these surfaces but between the penile dartos muscle and its subcutaneous tissues, specially adapted for this function.

Amputation of the foreskin considerably reduces or even totally destroys this mobility, by removing reserve of skin and eliminating this amazing function.

The effects of this loss may be slight if the man is a premature ejaculator, since the very brief intercourse will not cause irritation. The same may hold if the penis is very short or moved by thrusts of small amplitude. On the other hand, prolonged and vigorous intercourse with a circumcised penis risks causing irritation in spite of natural or even artificial lubrication. This explains certain cases of female and even male dyspareunia. I have examined a young man circumcised during military service whose erection was painful due to the sheer stretching of the remnant sheath. It had been cut too short over the erect corpora cavernosa. His sexual capacity, as a result, was, at least for a while, totally destroyed, and certainly altered for the rest of his life.

We may also question whether circumcision, so common in the United States, may be a factor encouraging erosions of the ano-rectal mucosa during anal intercourse, and may thus encourage the spread of HIV. As such, circumcision could be a crucial factor in the alarmingly and disproportionately high rate of HIV infection of the United States, since we know that breaks in the skin or mucosa are the usual portals of entry of the virus.

9.   CONCLUSION

It would appear, then, that resistance of the preputial orifice to premature retraction, which is normal and useful in infancy, diminishes in frequency with age due to the increasingly frequent manipulations of the penis. It depends, therefore, on the practice of masturbation, which permits an organized morphological development in the direction of future adult sexual behavior.

In those cases where the manipulation of the penis does not lead to permanent widening of the ring of the foreskin, this part remains of insufficient diameter to expose the glans and constitutes primary preputial stenosis ("phimosis") of the adolescent.

Prescription of kinestherapy is effective in widening this ring, and redirects the patient towards conventional masturbation. Resolution of the preputial stenosis can be achieved in a few weeks.

Tackling the subject of masturbation contributes to removing guilt from a very widespread genital activity, but one that is often very poorly accepted due to taboo, which continues without logic or reason.

In the absence of a cutaneous abnormality, manual remodeling of the foreskin seems always to be always effective. Medical treatment of adolescent preputial stenosis avoids all of the problems caused by amputation of the foreskin. Following circumcision, the cutaneous mobility of the penile sheath, being unable to benefit from the reserve of tissue, is restricted, and the dynamics of coitus are altered. In North America where circumcision is widespread, techniques to re-cover the glans by plastic surgery or stretching have been developed.[10] This latter method, by stretching the remaining skin, restores the mobility of the sheath almost as it would have been prior to the ablation.

We can be happy that directed and therapeutic manipulation of the foreskin allows the avoidance of surgical intervention and spares the patient from all of the unavoidable problems and disadvantages that result when surgery has occurred.

REFERENCES

1. Mendel G. Anthropologie Differentielle. Paris: Payot, 1972. p. 133. [...si on rappelle l'universalité de la masturbation infantile Durant les premières années, et sa quasi-universalité à l'adolescence chez le garçon, on reconnaît alors quelle place elle doit occuper.]
2. Freud S. La Naissance de la psychanalyse [Texte imprimé][aus den Anfänger der Psychoanalyse], lettres à Wilhelm Fliess, notes et plans, 1887-1902, publiées par Marie Bonaparte, Anna Freud, Ernst Kris. Traduit de l'allemand par Anne Berman. 2e édition.

Paris: Presses Universitaires de France, 1969. pp. 211-2, Cited in: Mendel G.. Anthropologie Differentielle. Paris: Payot, 1972. p. 133.

3. Mendel G. Anthropologie Differentielle. Paris: Payot, 1972. pp. 100. [En effet, auto-érotisme et activité fantasmatique sont conçus par nous comme des productions de même nature, c'est-à-dire de nature mnémonique, associative, secondaire.]

4. Mendel G. Anthropologie Differentielle. Paris: Payot, 1972. p. 120. [La masturbation n'est, en dernier ressort, que le moyen de raviver, de renouveler intensément, le souvenit du plaisir d'organe + le souvenit des multiples mnésies sensitivo-sensorielles qui constituent, lorsque stimulées, le fantasme.]

5. Mureau MA, Slijper FM, van der Meulen JC, Verhulst FC, Slob AK. Psychosexual adjustment of men who underwent hypospadias repair: a norm-related study. J Urol 1995 Oct;154(4):1351-5.

6. Taylor JR, Lockwood AP, Taylor AJ. The prepuce: specialized mucosa of the penis and its loss to circumcision. Br J Urol 1996 Feb;77(2):291-5.

7. Cold CJ, Taylor JR. The prepuce. BJU Int 1999 Jan;83 Suppl 1:34-44.

8. Fink KS, Carson CC, DeVellis RF. Adult circumcision outcomes study: effect on erectile function, penile sensitivity, sexual activity and satisfaction. J Urol 2002 May;167(5):2113-6.

9. Zwang G. La circoncision, pourquoir faire? Contraception, Fertilité, Sexualité 1977;5(3):247-53.

10. Bigelow J. The Joy of Uncircumcising! 2nd edition. Aptos, CA: Hourglass. 1995.

Chapter 6

PENILE TORTS IN THE COURTS

David Llewellyn, JD
Attorney at Law, Atlanta and Conyers, Georgia, USA

Abstract: As parents and young men become more aware of their rights, an increasing number of circumcision-related lawsuits have been filed. In the past, these suits have not always fared well in the courts but the situation seems to be changing in the United States and in other English-speaking countries. Young men for the first time are suing for damage done to them as infants. New theories of law are being advanced and old ones are being dusted off, although the success of these theories remains to be seen. What is the prospect for the future of genital injury litigation as the public becomes more aware of the damage caused by circumcision?

Key words: Circumcision, medical ethics, law

Today, just a few moments ago, in a nearby hospital maternity ward little Toby Smith,[1] a two-day old baby boy, was taken by a nurse from his mother's arms and breast. The nurse took him to the circumcision room of the hospital nursery where she stripped him naked from the waist down. She placed him on a cold, hard plastic Circumstraint™ board and bound his arms and legs with Velcro™ strips. Then she scrubbed his penis and scrotum with an antiseptic solution, thereby giving him an immediate erection. She put a drape across him, leaving his penis exposed through a hole in the cloth. He remained strapped in this position, scared, cold, crying, and unable to move, until it came his turn to be circumcised. Then the doctor came in. He was whistling because he has the afternoon off and has already planned a golf game with some of his fellow obstetricians at a local club. He has five circumcisions to do. Toby's is first.

Once the doctor began the circumcision, Toby underwent a lengthy period of excruciating pain. First, the doctor tore Toby's foreskin from his glans, using forceps or a blunt probe. This was necessary because the

Flesh and Blood, Edited by Denniston et al.
Kluwer Academic/Plenum Publishers, New York 2004

foreskin is bonded at birth to the glans penis by a shared common epithelial tissue. This connecting *synechia* must be broken before the circumcision can be done. The tearing caused Toby intense pain, and he began to scream. The doctor then used a hemostat to crush Toby's foreskin on the dorsal side, increasing his pain. Next, the circumciser used surgical scissors to make a cut the length of Toby's foreskin on the dorsal side, causing him even more pain, to which he reacted with a stronger cry that rose to a fit of screaming. The circumciser retracted Toby's foreskin; placed a 1.3 metal Gomco™ bell over his exposed glans; and pulled the foreskin forward up the length of the shaft over the bell.

Second, while Toby strained against the Velcro™ straps holding him down, the doctor placed the bottom portion of the Gomco™ clamp over the bell; applied the top portion of the clamp to the shaft of the bell; and closed the clamp, thus crushing the foreskin against the bell and causing Toby intense pain. His screaming increased, together with his heartbeat, cortisol level, and respiration rate, ultimately reaching measures of distress consistent with the torture that the doctor was inflicting upon him.

Third, the doctor cut off Toby's foreskin with a scalpel. Finally, the clamp was left in place for several minutes before it was removed. The entire procedure took *at least* five minutes, and probably more, and was done without any anesthesia whatsoever.

Immediately after the circumcision, Toby's glans penis and foreskin remnant were raw, red, and extremely painful to touch. In order to protect Toby's penis from further damage, the doctor placed Vaseline™ on a pad of gauze and placed it over the penis. At this point, Toby was whimpering and quivering, and was most likely in clinical shock.

As a result of his circumcision, Toby will continue to suffer pain for at least two weeks while the wound heals. Every time he urinates or is changed, he will feel pain and will cry. He will become fussy, whereas before he had been a normal, calm baby boy. This fussiness will interfere with normal infant/maternal bonding.

Moreover, Toby suffered a permanent deformity due to the loss of a normal, healthy body part that is a normal part of male anatomy. He lost the protective covering of the glans penis with the result that, throughout his life, he has greater risk of damage to his glans from burns and other injuries. In addition, sexual activity when he is an adult and is married will be more difficult than had he not been circumcised. He permanently lost a significant percentage of his penile skin, been deprived of having normal sexual intercourse, and been deprived of having the sensations that are provided by the nerve endings in the inner lining of the foreskin during intercourse. Over the coming years, as a result of his circumcision, Toby will be subjected to cornification (callousing) of the glans of his penis with a resulting loss of sensitivity. In the event of exposure to certain venereal diseases, his risk of contracting them will be more likely, rather than less likely. He will be more susceptible to pain from other sources, and will feel other pain more intensely because his pain threshold has been permanently lowered. Further, he will be subject to contracting meatitis, inflammation of the meatus (urinary opening) of the glans penis. Recurrent meatitis and loss of the frenular artery, which is usually destroyed during a Gomco™ circumcision, have both been linked with an increased incidence of meatal stenosis, a narrowing of the urinary opening, which often requires surgical correction. Further, thanks to his mother's doctor, Toby is now at risk for the re-adherence of the foreskin remnant to the glans, forming a skin bridge or tunnel that will make sexual intercourse as well as cleanliness more difficult, and often requires surgical correction.

This is the reality of neonatal male circumcision. Even a properly performed circumcision has serious consequences for its victim. However, circumcisions often are done without permission. Sometimes things go wrong and the child is badly injured beyond the harm of the circumcision itself. What legal remedies does the child have? When must these be exercised? How are circumcision suits faring in the courts?

I am an attorney at law who concentrates his practice in the area of civil litigation. Since becoming involved in a wrongful circumcision case in 1995 in Alabama, genital injury litigation has become an increasingly large percentage of my practice. Although we are far from the general acceptance by the courts of the rather simple proposition that all circumcisions on non-consenting minors are criminal assaults unless performed for immediate therapeutic reasons, it does appear that the courts are increasingly receptive to circumcision lawsuits. In addition, the interest by the general public in bringing circumcision lawsuits has increased dramatically.

At present, there are four generally recognized causes of action for the most common penile torts. The first of these is the tort of battery. Generally, any offensive touching of one person by another without the consent of the person touched constitutes the tort of battery. Therefore, the circumcision of an infant or child without the consent of at least one parent gives rise to liability for battery in most American states. From the number of cases in which I have been involved during the last seven years, it appears that this tort is extremely common. Since 1995, I have represented or am in the process of representing fourteen individuals, thirteen children and one adult, who were circumcised without consent. Just this week, another attorney has consulted me about associating on a fifteenth case. Prior to the 1990s, these cases were somewhat rare. Perhaps this was because of the lack of damages awarded by the courts. Indeed, the legal literature is bereft of reports of recoveries for circumcision without consent.[2] However, beginning early in the last decade, the tide appeared to turn. In the early 1990s, in *Ruiz-Castillo v. Kaiser Permanente Hospital,* Santa Clara Superior Court, California, No.

648925, filed by my colleague Charles Bonner, the plaintiff obtained a $60,000 settlement for being wrongfully circumcised. In *Brown v. Jackson Hospital and Clinic*, Circuit Court of Montgomery County, Alabama, No. CV92-1929, the first case in which I was involved, a jury in 1995 awarded the minor plaintiff $65,000, including $55,000 for future damages. Since then, I have settled numerous cases for significant sums. It is apparent now that wrongful circumcision cases finally have significant value. Of course, I hope that by plaintiffs' bringing every possible wrongful circumcision case, doctors will soon become aware that they must be very careful in obtaining consent and that these cases will soon cease to be the common source of litigation that they are today.

In addition, while not directly related to circumcision, the forcible retraction of a boy's foreskin without the permission of his parent is generally a battery. To my knowledge, there are no cases reported in the legal literature involving forcible retraction. Heretofore, the only case of which I had knowledge was one brought in a small claims court in the State of Washington, which resulted in a verdict for $100. This may soon change. In February, 2002, I filed the case of *Robertson v. Fayette Medical Clinic, P.C.,* Civil Action File No. 2002 V 0150 CE, in the Superior Court of Fayette County, Georgia. There, a young mother alleges that, when the defendant physician examined her intact son, who had a somewhat short foreskin and a mild hypospadias, he forcibly retracted the foreskin and tore it from the glans. Thereafter, the foreskin was so short, the child suffered from balanoposthitis on a regular basis because feces became trapped between his foreskin and glans. My client and I hope this case will not only result in an appropriate monetary award but also will enlighten the doctor and the court concerning pain of forcible retraction and the very real harm to a boy caused by it.

General negligence in the performance of medical services, usually called medical malpractice, is the second cause of action commonly used to vindicate circumcision injuries. While the most devastating injuries, such as complete penile ablation, have always been compensable, until recently, penile injuries due to circumcision seem to have been given little consideration by the courts. For example, in the cases of *Kadel v. Zlotnik, Case No. 674324* in the Superior Court for San Diego County, California, a jury, on 31 October 1994, awarded only $36,400 to a boy who sued his circumciser for cutting off a portion of the tip of his penis during a neonatal circumcision. Such an award seems clearly inadequate. However, more recent cases give us hope. In *Clark v. Lu*, in the Kankakee Illinois Circuit Court, a jury in 1997 awarded $327,749 to an infant who suffered removal of too much skin during a circumcision, an injury made worse by a second surgeon. The *New England Jury Verdict Review & Analysis* in 1999 reported on a Massachusetts case in which a child who had suffered the severing of a three millimeter portion from the tip of his glans penis, which was thereafter successfully reattached, settled his suit against the circumcising physician for a structured settlement with a present value of $500,000. In 1999, an Australian man finally recovered over Aus$360,000 for a botched circumcision at birth that had removed most of his penile shaft skin.[3] Earlier this year, I settled a case for the sum of $300,000 for a Georgia boy who lost a small portion of his ventral glans, including his corona from approximately three o'clock to nine o'clock, during a routine circumcision. In short, it appears that the prospect for reasonable recoveries for non-catastrophic, yet significant, penile injuries due to circumcision are increasing. I expect that, as more parents become aware of circumcision damage issues, these cases will increase in number.

Also, under the heading of negligence, may be found those cases in which parents consent to circumcision without being informed as to its risks and disadvantages, later find out the truth, and then sue on behalf of the child, claiming a lack of informed consent. The legal doctrine of informed consent states that, in order for a physician to obtain legal consent to surgery, he or she must inform the person giving consent of all the generally accepted risks and disadvantages of a surgery that a reasonable person would want to know. If the physician fails to so inform a patient and a reasonable patient would not have undergone the surgery if fully informed, then a cause of action for lack of informed consent, as medical malpractice or medical negligence, exists. To my knowledge no such suit in regard to circumcision has ever been successful. However, that principle is presently being tested in the case of *Flatt v. Kantak*, District Court of Cass County, North Dakota, Civil Action No. 99-3761, in which my colleague Zenas Baer represents the plaintiffs. It is hoped that this case will establish once and for all the principle that merely asking if one desires circumcision or not for one's son is not sufficient to meet the requirements of informed consent. If *Flatt* results in a recovery for the plaintiffs, I would expect that many more such suits will be filed in the future, including suits by young men when they reach the age of majority.

The other cause of action generally available in regard to circumcision is the equitable remedy of injunction. This is most often used when parents cannot agree whether or not to circumcise the child. In the past four years, I have been actively involved in three such cases, all of which were resolved either by dismissal or by agreement of the parties. The lesson to be learned from these cases is that a suit for injunctive relief, while onerous and expensive, can save the child from an unnecessary circumcision. Unfortunately, it will be some time before such cases entirely disappear. For example, only this week I have been consulted by a young unmarried mother who is concerned that the father of her baby may attempt to have the child circumcised against her wishes while exercising his visitation rights with the child.

In summary, battery, negligence either in the performance of the surgery or in the obtaining of consent, and injunctive relief are traditional causes of action that are being used with increasing success in the genital injury area. However, new theoretical developments in the law are creating the possibility of expanding those causes of action. Within the last ten years, an increasing body of legal literature has questioned whether or not the circumcision of a healthy boy is legal at all.

Perhaps the earliest legal commentator to question the legality of neonatal circumcision was William E. Brigman. In the mid-1980s, he concluded: "Since circumcision is medically unwarranted mutilation and disfigurement, it would appear to be a clear case of child abuse."[4] The legal literature in this country thereafter remained remarkably silent until a law student in 1997 published a law review note criticizing the United States' outlawing of female circumcision while continuing to allow infant male circumcision. In "Justifying the Unjustifiable: Rite v. Wrong," Abbie J. Chessler came to the conclusion that, "regardless of whether a child is male or female, neither should be subject to genital mutilation. The United States' criticism of other cultures and religions is self-righteous and ironic, especially since it continues to advocate its own abusive ritual based on unsound medical justifications."[5] It is unfortunate that a similar cogent argument was not accepted by the United States Court of Appeals for the 8th Circuit, which in 1997 rejected an equal protection attack upon North Dakota's female genital mutilation statute by finding that the plaintiffs lacked standing to bring the suit. See *Fishbeck v. State of North Dakota*, 115 F.3d 580 (8th Cir. 1997).

Chessler's remarkable article was followed shortly by another in which another law student, Ross Povenmire, concluded that parents did not have the legal authority to consent to neonatal circumcision. While recognizing that "in the United States, parents are presumed to have the power to consent to this circumcision of their infant sons," he concluded that the "practice is no longer tenable given the emerging recognition of constitutional rights for minors, the ambiguous and highly qualified status of parental interests in medical decision making on behalf of children, and the important state interest in insuring the protection of children's health."[6] Thereafter, another article in the medical literature suggested that existing child abuse laws and other medical principles may give rise to liability on the part of a physician who routinely circumcises an infant boy.[7] At the same time, another law student questioned once again whether or not the criminalization of female circumcision in the United States violated the equal protection clause of the Fourteenth Amendment to the Constitution by only protecting females.[8]

Then, in the last year of the old millennium, a flurry of articles continued to question the legality of neonatal circumcision. The first, an Australian article, opined that "[g]iven international instruments and domestic common law principles in case law, grave doubt exists as to whether a truly informed parent can consent to the non-therapeutic circumcision of the child."[9] This article was quickly followed by another in the American literature that concluded that, "because routine circumcision causes significant harm while providing no appreciable medical benefits, parental consent to the procedure is invalid. If circumcision can ever ethically and legally be performed, it is only when the male reaches adulthood and is capable of deciding for himself to undergo the procedure."[10] That year also saw the publication of a similar article by another law student, Matthew R. Giannetti, who suggested that the American Academy of Pediatrics might be subject to trade association liability for promoting needless neonatal circumcision by reason of its negligent or intentional provision to the consuming public of misrepresentations of significant information regarding the risks, effects, and purported benefits of that surgery.[11]

Finally, this year has seen the publication of yet another article that concludes that routine neonatal circumcision is medically unethical in that it "fails to satisfy the criteria necessary to justify it either as a public health measure or a procedure performed in the best interest of the individual. The human rights burden posed to the individual is severe and is not outweighed by any appreciable public health gain."[12] In addition, in Canada, the Registrar of the College of Physician and Surgeons of Saskatchewan has recently warned its members that they should seek legal counsel if they intend to continue circumcising infants in view of the lack of medical justification for the procedure.[13] In short, there now exists a substantial body of legal and medical literature that suggests strongly, if it does not prove unequivocally, that neonatal male circumcision as practiced in the United States can never be justified and is tortious misconduct under generally accepted principles of Anglo-American tort law.

Legal commentary, however, does not necessarily guarantee success in the courts. As anyone who has studied the history of the United States' civil rights movement knows, theory does not always equal practice. This is especially true in the context of a surgery that, in the past, was performed so often that it still seems to many no more significant than the cutting of the umbilical cord at birth and one that has psycho-sexual, as well as religious, overtones. Nevertheless, this theoretical framework can now be used to press forward with valid cases that will test the limits of the law.

One recent development, which I believe has arisen directly from the publicity that the National Organization of Circumcision Information Resource Centers (NOCIRC) and other individuals and groups have given to the issue of neonatal circumcision is that young men are finally coming forward and complaining that what was done to them as newborns was wrong. One such young man is William Stowell. At the age of fourteen William discovered that he was circumcised. After doing considerable research on his own, he came to the conclusion that he had been needlessly harmed as a baby. He decided to do something about it as soon as he legally could. When he became eighteen, he consulted me for legal assistance. I agreed to assist in seeing what could be done legally about his circumcision performed eighteen years earlier. His mother had not wanted to have him circumcised, but he had come home from the hospital circumcised anyway. When we retrieved the medical records, we discovered a consent form signed by his mother. However, we also discovered that when she signed the consent form she was under the influence of painkillers that altered her mental status and also was suffering from the effects of delivery by Cesarean section the day before. She did not recall signing the form, and had not wanted to do so. Therefore, William filed suit against his circumciser in the United States District Court for the Eastern District of New York in December 2000, just before he became nineteen years of age.[14] The defendants immediately filed motions to dismiss, claiming that the case sounded in medical malpractice, which was barred by a ten-year statute of limitation that was not tolled while William was a minor. We argued that, because consent obtained from a person who is intoxicated is no consent at all, the case sounded in the tort of battery, which was what we had pleaded, among other causes of action, all of which were not yet barred by a statute of limitation because the applicable statutes of limitation were tolled during his minority. In the autumn of last year, the District Court denied the motions to dismiss. The case is presently proceeding to the discovery phase.

Williams' case is the first I know of that has been brought to attack a routinely performed circumcision eighteen years after the fact, when the only damage was the circumcision itself and its usual deleterious effects. However, it is based upon sound legal principles, which we believe we will be able to prove. It is novel only in the sense that such a case has not been brought before. It has attracted tremendous attention from the media. Shortly after it was filed, it was the subject of an on-line article by *Newsweek Magazine*. Early last year, William and I were interviewed by Charles Gibson on ABC's *Good Morning America*. I have been interviewed concerning the case by radio stations from Los Angeles to Detroit to Columbus, Ohio, to the country of Columbia. In its December 2001 issue, the case was the subject of the "Penis Page" in *Penthouse Magazine*. It has raised the public's consciousness about the very real ethical and legal issues surrounding neonatal circumcision.

I trust that William's brave stance is only the beginning of a number of lawsuits that will establish once and for all exactly what the legal commentators have been saying: Routine neonatal circumcision by doctors is illegal and its performance constitutes at least the tort of battery. Presently, I have been consulted by a nineteen-year-old young man who is considering suing his circumciser. His case is different in that his parents willingly consented to the circumcision. However, the only reason they did so was so that he would look like his father. If he decides to bring suit, he will claim that such consent was invalid because no parent may consent to cosmetic surgery on the normal, non-deformed body part of a minor. It is clear to me that circumcision is no more than social scarring or a modern day tribal marking. If a father allowed a physician to scarify his son's face so as to make the boy look like the father, who had also been scarified by his father, no court would have difficulty in finding that a tort had been committed by the operating physician. Likewise, in a case where a father decides for his son to be circumcised merely so that the son "will look like Dad," the tort is no less egregious. In each case, the motivation is precisely the same. Therefore, the illegality of both should be obvious to any thoughtful, non-biased court.

In the future, I believe that we can expect to see numerous suits by young men who finally come to the realization that they have been unjustly damaged as infants. These cases will probably, at first, seem shocking to the public. Eventually, however, they will be accepted because they will be based upon sound legal precedent and principle. In the end, I believe they will be very effective in wearing down the medical profession's enthusiasm for making money at the expense of little boys' penises and their future sexual happiness.

What else does the future hold? I believe that Matthew Gianetti's article, suggesting that the American Academy of Pediatrics be held liable under the doctrine of trade association liability for the negligent provision of erroneous or incomplete information, points the way to eventually forcing that organization to confront honestly the medical literature. The Association's two latest circumcision statements, I believe, were justly criticized by Mr. Gianetti for their significant omissions as well as their misstatements. However, the American Academy of Pediatrics is not alone in publishing trade association advice for the public that glosses over the harm of circumcision and completely ignores the important functions of the foreskin. Other trade associations such as the American Academy of Family Practice and the American College of Obstetricians and Gynecologists may also find themselves the subjects of lawsuits if they do not quickly reform their literature so as to conform to the full truth.

Finally, numerous persons have suggested to me that a class action lawsuit might bring an end to neonatal circumcision. While I cannot say that there is a single class action lawsuit that will have that effect, I believe that individual hospitals may possibly be subject to class actions for allowing cosmetic surgery on infants in their facilities or for pushing circumcision for their own financial advantage. For example, Northside Hospital in Atlanta, Georgia, in 1995, was still using a Discharge Summary Sheet, which said on it "Circumcision Status: No circumcision _____ Reason _____," followed by "No Bleeding _____ Vaseline Gauze Applied _____." This form clearly required the discharging nurse to note any newborn male who left the hospital intact and to demand a reason at least from one parent for the decision to leave the child as God and nature made him. Such pressure by hospitals, which is well-known but little discussed, may very well give rise to a class action lawsuit on behalf of himself and others by an infant whose parents were talked into circumcision at the last moment by an overly aggressive nurse or physician. At the very least, such a form is evidence of a pro-circumcision bias that leads to unnecessary cosmetic surgery on infants. Since a hospital has a duty to protect those in its care, it is only a matter of time before a court correctly recognizes that for a hospital to allow needless cosmetic surgery on the penis of an infant merely to satisfy the parents' desires is as much a tort as it would be to allow the application of tribal scars to the child's cheeks or to permit the clitoridectomy of a baby girl to satisfy her parents' notion of female beauty.

Last, but not least, there is the possibility of a class action suit against any Roman Catholic hospital that has permitted the non-therapeutic circumcision of male infants since the publication of the most recent Catholic Catechism. A brave activist, Petrina Fadel, wrote me recently that she has sent letters to 171 Roman Catholic bishops and cardinals in the United States, as well as one to the Pope,[15] in which she pointed out that, because the Catechism of the Catholic Church states, "[e]xcept when performed for strictly therapeutic medical reasons, directly intended amputations, mutilations, and sterilizations performed on innocent persons are against the moral law," and, because routine male circumcision is clearly an amputation and is not done "for strictly therapeutic medical reasons," the performance of circumcision on children violates Catholic doctrine. It is only a matter of time until a Catholic youth claims the protection of the doctrine of the Church and sues the Catholic hospital where he was circumcised on behalf of himself and all others similarly situated for failure to protect him from the amputation and mutilation from which he should be free, according to Church law.

In short, suits regarding circumcision are only in their infancy. As long as the American medical profession continues down its path of permitting social surgery on infants, it will be liable to attack in the courts by children as they reach the age of majority. The legal attack on circumcision has "not yet begun to fight."[16]

EDITORS NOTE

Since the presentation of this paper, the William Stowell case was settled out of court and William Haynes became the second eighteen-year-old male to file a lawsuit against the doctor and hospital for having circumcised him.

REFERENCES

1. "Toby Smith" and his circumcision are fictional; but the acts and suffering they portray are everyday realities in most United States hospitals.
2. In fact, I have only been able to find two such cases. In <u>Noe v. Kaiser Foundation Hospitals</u>, 435 P.2d 306 (Or. 1967) an award of punitive damages for unauthorized circumcision was reversed. The case did not recite the amount awarded for compensatory damages. In <u>Kalina v. General Hospital of City of Syracuse</u>, 31 Misc.2d 18, 22 N.Y.S.2d 733, *aff'd* 18 A.D.2d 757, 235 N.Y.S.2d 808 (4th Dept. 1962), *aff'd* 13 N.Y.2d 1023, 245 N.Y.S.2d 599, 195 N.E.2d 309 (Ct App. 1963), the court denied the parents of a Jewish child the right to recover damages for themselves because their child was circumcised by a doctor in the hospital rather than being ritually circumcised on his 8th day by a mohel.
3. Peterson, SE Assaulted and mutilated: a personal account of circumcision trauma. In Denniston, GC, Hodges FM, Milos, MF, editors. Understanding Circumcision: A Multi-Disciplinary Approach to a Multi-Dimensional Problem. New York: Kluwer Academic/Plenum Publishers; 2001. pp. 271-289.
4. Brigman, WE. Circumcision as child abuse: the legal and constitutional issues. J. Fam. L. (1984-85), 23.3: 337-357, 342.
5. Chessler, A. J. Justifying the unjustifiable: rite v. wrong. Buffalo L. Rev. (1997), 45: 555-613, 612.
6. Povenmire, R. Do parents have the legal authority to consent to the surgical amputation of normal, healthy tissue from their infant children?: the practice of circumcision in the United States. J. Gen., Soc. Pol. & L. (1988-1999), 7,1: 187-122, 106.
7. Van Howe, RS., Svoboda, JS, Dwyer, JG, Price, CP. Involuntary circumcision: the legal issues. B.J.U. International (1999), 83. Suppl. 1: 63-73.
8. Bond, SL. State laws criminalizing female circumcision: a violation of the equal protection clause of the fourteenth amendment?, J. Mar. L. Rev. (1999) 32.2: 353-380.
9. Boyle, GJ, Svoboda, JS, Price, CP, Turner, JN. Circumcision of healthy boys, criminal assault?. J. L. & Med. (2000), 7: 301-310, 309 (footnote omitted).
10. Svoboda, J. S, Van Howe, RS, Dwyer, JG. Informed consent for neonatal circumcision: an ethical and legal conundrum. J Contemp. Health L. & Pol. (2000), 17: 61-133, 62-63.
11. Giannetti, MR. Circumcision and the American Academy of Pediatrics: should scientific misconduct result in trade association liability? Iowa L. Rev. (May 2000), 85.4: 1507-1568.
12. Hodges, FM, Svoboda, JS, Van Howe, RS. Prophylactic interventions on children: balancing human rights with public health, J. Med. Ethics (2002) 28: 10-16, 15.
13. Kendel, DA, Caution against routine circumcision of newborn male infants. Memorandum to the members of the College of Physicians and Surgeons of Saskatchewan, Canada (February 20,2002). www.intact.ca/saskmemo.html (accessed April 3, 2002).
14. <u>Stowell v. Good Samaritan Hospital,</u> C.A. File No. CV007501, U.S.D.C., E.D.N.Y.
15. Private electronic communication dated April 1, 2002.
16. With apologies to the United States' naval hero John Paul Jones.

Chapter 7

THE ACTIVIST'S RIGHTS IN THE WORKPLACE

Charles Bonner, JD
Attorney at Law, Sausalito, California

Abstract: This paper focuses on recent successful legal strategies for challenging workplace discrimination on the basis of political views, cultural bias, and lack of awareness to the constitutional right of children to bodily integrity. It covers a case study involving a human rights activist who sought to educate and elevate the awareness of co-workers to the legal rights of the child to an intact body.

Key words: Circumcision, law, US constitution, gender discrimination

When a young military man named William Stowell decided to talk to high school students about how he had been circumcised at birth without his consent and how he had sued the hospital where this abuse of his right to autonomy and bodily integrity had occurred,[1-2] he was probably unaware that he was doing something momentous.

When Rosa Parks sat in that infamous public bus in Montgomery, Alabama, she decided that she would disregard an unjust law that required her to move to the back of the bus because of the color of her skin. She was not intending to advance the cause of civil rights. She did not know at the time that she would light the torch of universal human rights that would become a beacon for the whole world to follow toward freedom. Martin Luther King was probably unaware that he was doing something of universal and permanent significance when he proclaimed his dream of freedom, equality, and human rights, not just for disenfranchised African-Americans but for everyone in the world. He would never have predicted that his life and contributions would be memorialized with a national holiday.

I submit to you that, as we come together from around the globe to protect the rights of children all over the world, we are doing something important; something that will have an extraordinarily powerful positive impact on millions of children around the world.

I have been involved in the movement to protect the rights of infants and children to bodily integrity for over sixteen years. Primarily, I have accomplished this by suing doctors. David Llewellyn, Zenas Baer, and I are among the few lawyers who are challenging the medical profession to improve its human rights record and to cease its habitual violation of basic principles of medical ethics.

Recently, however, my work has branched in a new direction. Employees in medical and non-medical industries have been contacting me for advice about their civil rights in the workplace regarding advocating against routine infant circumcision. In fact, a person at this symposium approached me and said: I have been trying to contact you. My employers are trying to fire me because I am advocating for the rights of the child. Indeed, this movement gained momentum some twenty years ago when Marilyn Milos was discriminated against in the workplace for educating parents about the facts pertaining to circumcision and for informing them that they had the power to protect their newborn boys from unnecessary surgery.

Because of this groundswell of public demand for legal redress against discrimination in the workplace, I have now augmented the list of target defendants to include employers who attempt to prohibit, forbid, or curtail the freedom of concerned citizens to advocate publicly on behalf of the rights of the child.

Recently, I settled a case for a client against one of the largest national banks in the nation. A vice-president of the bank, my client, was a very productive hard-working man who had received numerous awards and cash bonuses. His work was exemplary during his four-and-a-half-year tenure with the bank until the day he loaned a pregnant co-worker the award-winning documentary film, *Whose Body, Whose Rights?*, a film that had been repeatedly broadcast on PBS television stations across the nation. My client's co-worker knew the film focused on the infant male circumcision controversy, knew the film had recently been broadcast on her local PBS station, and knew my client was interviewed in the film. She accepted the film and took it home to watch with her husband. The bank's sexual harassment investigator called my client into her office, chastised him for engaging in offensive sexual conduct, and accused him of circulating a sexually explicit film that showed an actual circumcision in all its bloody detail. She informed him that she was recommending his termination. Indeed, the bank terminated him immediately.

We then sued the bank along with the manager who initiated my client's termination. The bank took a "scorched earth" approach to this litigation. They threw every imaginable motion at us, trying to have the lawsuit thrown out of court.

As part of our legal strategy, we were able to develop a number of novel theories. For instance, we argued that the bank was illegally attempting to prohibit an employee from expressing his political views in the workplace. We had clear evidence that this actually occurred in my client's case. His boss had openly said to him: What were you thinking? You had to know when you gave her this video that you were on the wrong side of this issue! When we stated that the bank was illegally interfering with my client's right to express a political view, the bank countered: We can terminate him at will. We have that right. The bank relied on a law passed during the Civil War that prohibits a bank vice president from suing his employers. The National Banking Act was passed in 1864 to improve the sale of Civil War bonds. Every other bank vice president who has sued his employer since 1864 has had his case thrown out without being heard because of that antiquated law.

We also charged the bank with breach of contract. Everyone has a contractual right to work in a discrimination-free environment. Additionally, we charged the bank with a breach of the covenant of good faith and fair dealing. Every contract has in it a legally imposed covenant that each party to the contract will deal with each other fairly and in good faith with respect to the performance of the contract.

The bank spent well in excess of one million dollars litigating this case. Nevertheless, we fought our way through the courts, and we won. The bank appealed, but we also won on appeal. We now have restored the civil rights of some one hundred thousand (100,000) American bank vice-presidents who previously were without legal recourse.

In California, the law provides that an employer cannot restrict, coerce, or otherwise interfere with an employee's right to engage in political activity. If there is any state or country that does not have that law, I suggest you advocate to establish such an important law. My client's case was the first case in which a view about male circumcision was rightly considered a political view. Its status as a genuine political view is obvious because we already have laws in this country outlawing female circumcision. We do not yet have a similar law outlawing male circumcision. This is a political issue of discrimination on the basis of gender, in violation of federal and state civil rights laws that must be reckoned with.

We learned a number of things from this case that may help other political activists in the workplace. First, companies fear any association with a particular point of political view. They want to know whether an employee is an activist, and, if so, they want to know for what cause. They will permit an employee to work on a cause, and they will allow the employee to reveal where he works, but they insist that the employee state that his views are not necessarily those of his company.

Second, there are other claims that one can bring cases such as wrongful discipline and public policy. In the United States, whenever employers discriminate against employees, they violate the public policy that the workplace is to be free from discrimination. In California, you can bring an individual tort (a civil wrong) claim solely for violation of public policy without claims of discrimination. In other words, if there are no facts evidencing discrimination on the basis of protected classifications, such as race, religion, national origin, gender, sexual preference, etc., a claim for violation of public policy could still be advanced.

Third, another claim that can be brought against employers who attempt to deny employees the right to express political views is the intentional infliction of emotional distress. Employers engaging in extreme and outrageous conduct that should not be tolerated by a civilized society are liable for the tort of intentional infliction of emotional distress and punitive damages. Discrimination, for example, is extreme and outrageous conduct.

If you have a situation where a boy's penis is being cut, and the employer refuses to allow the employee to voice his protest, the employer may be guilty of creating a hostile working environment. Cutting a boy's penis is severe conduct. If you tell the employee that he cannot speak against this conduct, then the employer is said to be retaliating against that employee.

Retaliation exists when three things occur: (1) There is some adverse employment action taken against an employee; (2) the employee is engaging in a protected activity; and (3) there is a temporal proximity between the political activity and the retaliatory conduct.

If an employee, for instance, expresses the view that a boy's penis should be protected from routine infant circumcision, that employee is engaging in a protected political activity. He is advocating on behalf of the boy. If the employer disciplines the employee through suspension, termination, or otherwise for the employee's advocacy on behalf of the child, the employer's action may be illegal retaliation.

A recent case of mine illustrates this point. An African-American law enforcement agent was protesting racist comments made against Jews by his co-workers. He expressed the view that it was wrong to call Jews offensive names. His employer retaliated against him by repeatedly refusing to promote him. Corporate counsel for the employer claimed that, since the African-American agent was not Jewish, he could not claim discrimination against Jews. This was a false assertion contrary to our laws. The beauty of our legal system is that it is based on the idea that All men [and women] are created equal, and they are endowed by their Creator with certain inalienable rights, among those the right to life, liberty, and the pursuit of happiness. Because these are God-given rights, any human being has the right to complain about any discrimination against any other human being. If you are retaliated against for protecting a child, a Catholic, a Jew, an African-

American, or a European-American, then you are engaging in protected activity. If your employer takes adverse action against you, you can bring a claim under discrimination laws, including a claim for retaliation.

Aside from the above potential claims that may be asserted on behalf of the activist in the workplace, if you look at almost any page of the Constitution of the United States, you will see how circumcision is a violation of the child's rights. Michael Kinane, Esq., and I wrote an article in 1989 about the rights of the child to be free from these unwarranted restraints and this lack of freedom.[3] The First Amendment, guaranteeing the right to freedom of religion, freedom of expression, states:

> Congress shall make no law respecting an establishment of religion, or prohibiting the free exercise thereof; or abridging the freedom of speech, or of the press; or the right of the people peaceably to assemble, and to petition the government for a redress of grievances.

Many of these fundamental principles perfectly correlate with the right to protection from routine infant circumcision. For valid religious reasons, many males would prefer to remain genitally intact if given a choice. Indiscriminate circumcision of any male, regardless of the religious tradition or lack thereof into which he is born, necessarily imposes the stigma of a particular religion (Judaism or Islam) on a male who might well reject that religion. This thereby impairs the free exercise of a person's own religion or his right to freedom from religion. An infant, circumcised without his consent, is necessarily deprived of this First Amendment protection of free religious expression, free speech, and the right to legally challenge by petitioning his government with a grievance against routine infant circumcision.

The Fourth Amendment, protecting the right to be free from unreasonable searches and seizures, states:

> The right of the people to be secure in their persons, houses, papers, and effects, against unreasonable searches and seizures, shall not be violated, and no warrants shall issue, but upon probable cause, supported by oath or affirmation, and particularly describing the place to be searched, and the persons or things to be seized.

This amendment is violated whenever a child is circumcised for the obvious reason that the child, and a part of the child's body has been seized and removed without probable cause, or warrant [court order] since there is no medical justification.

The practice of circumcision clearly violates the Fifth Amendment, which guarantees the right to due process and the right to life and property:

> No person shall be held to answer for a capital, or otherwise infamous crime, unless on a presentment or indictment of a grand jury, except in cases arising in the land or naval forces, or in the militia, when in actual service in time of war or public danger; nor shall any person be subject for the same offense to be twice put in jeopardy of life or limb; nor shall he be compelled in any criminal case to be a witness against himself, nor be deprived of life, liberty, or property, without due process of law; nor shall private property be taken for public use, without just compensation.

This amendment is violated because circumcision, like any surgical procedure, necessarily endangers the child's life and, most importantly, deprives him of a part of his own body.

The Sixth Amendment states:

> In all criminal prosecutions, the accused shall enjoy the right to a speedy and public trial, by an impartial jury of the state and district wherein the crime shall have been committed, which district shall have been previously ascertained by law, and to be informed of the nature and cause of the accusation; to be confronted with the witnesses against him; to have compulsory process for obtaining witnesses in his favor, and to have the assistance of counsel for his defense.

Circumcision clearly violates this important amendment because a child who is subjected to circumcision has been denied any representative to advocate his constitutional right to retain his body parts.

The Eighth Amendment reads:

> Excessive bail shall not be required, nor excessive fines imposed, nor cruel and unusual punishments inflicted.

This crucial right to protection from cruel and unusual punishment is clearly violated whenever a child is circumcised, especially when circumcised without any form of anesthesia or analgesia before, during, or after the circumcision. This child has committed no crime, yet he is subjected to a most egregious form of genital torture without any immediate medical necessity.

The second sentence of the first section of the Fourteenth Amendment states:

> No state shall make or enforce any law which shall abridge the privileges or immunities of citizens of the United States; nor shall any state deprive any person of life, liberty, or property, without due process of law; nor deny any person within its jurisdiction the equal protection of the laws.

This fundamental right to due process and equal protection is clearly violated whenever a boy is circumcised because in the United States girls are legally protected from circumcision.

As mentioned, discrimination laws are useful in cases based on violation of the United States Constitution. Recently, I won the right, by federal court order, to present a claim under the Fourteenth Amendment equal protection and due process provisions on behalf of a child who was circumcised at birth and his parents who had not consented to the circumcision. This case, taking place in Brooklyn, New York, involves a Hispanic mother and a Greek father, both of whom are from cultures where circumcision is not practiced. The hospital where the boy was circumcised routinely circumcised Hispanic boys by having the parents sign consent forms in English. In this case, the mother did not speak or read English and the father was not present when the consent was signed. This hospital routinely presents an English consent form to non-English speaking parents. The Judge has ruled in our favor that in my case, the parents may assert a Fourteenth Amendment Claim for denial of due process based on the lack of an informed consent to the circumcision; and the child may assert a Fourteenth Amendment Claim for denial of equal protection by being treated differently than children of English-speaking parents who can understand the English document of informed consent.

California law states that an employer shall not engage in an employment practice that will discriminate against an employee on the basis of certain identified classifications: race, gender, national origin, religion, and, in California but not in federal law, sexual preference. It is not essential to have a sexual preference law because there are numerous ways to creatively plead any kind of sexual orientation claim under gender discrimination law. For instance, every child has a constitutional right to an intact body. If females are guaranteed legal protection from violations of bodily integrity but males are denied this protection, then males are being discriminated against on the basis of gender. Discrimination against males, sadly, is common in our society. Every day, we read about child abuse in the newspapers. Every day, there is another priest, Boy Scout leader, or caregiver who is charged with molesting boys across the United States and the world. Imagine for a moment how much greater the reaction would be if the newspapers were instead reporting the abuse of girls on such an incredibly large scale. The public outcry would be much louder and effective remedies to stop the abuse would be immediately instituted. However, routine infant male circumcision, a clear form of child abuse, receives little or no reaction from the public around the world. The realization that this abuse is rampant should make us aware that we must redouble our efforts.

Most of us in this society are prisoners of misinformation and disinformation. I certainly am. When I saw my newborn son being strapped down on a circumcision board, with hands and feet secured as if he was being prepared for execution, and saw the doctor take a scalpel to my son's little penis, I almost passed out. Because I am genitally intact, I failed to understand why I was agreeing to do this. This experience dramatically shaped my views on the legal, ethical, and moral aspects of the circumcision controversy. I would support my son in a lawsuit against his physician. I would almost support him in a lawsuit against me. I should have known better even though my wife and I had unwittingly received pre-packaged disinformation that was heavily biased towards the interests of the doctor and the hospital.

In the workplace, as in the doctor's office, our views are shaped and our actions are directed by those who are biased toward circumcision. It is going to take time for this cultural paradigm shift to occur, but I am confident that it will occur. In the meantime, we must keep working toward that goal. Part of that work is to secure the rights of the employee to free expression of his political and ethical views in the workplace.

In closing, let me stress that now is the time to protect and defend our children. Circumcision is as much child abuse as beating and neglect. We need to guarantee the constitutional right to bodily integrity for every child.

REFERENCES

1. Kuntzman G. Sex life not good? Sue! Lawyer David Llewellyn is the Johnnie Cochran of the circumcised. Newsweek Web (February 26, 2001).
   URL: http://www.nocircnc.org/Newsweek.htm
2. Suing over circumcision: man says lack of foreskin hurts sex life. ABC News.com URL: http://abcnews.go.com/sections/GMA/GoodMorningAmerica/GMA010207Circumcision_Suit.html [access date: 4 July 2002].
3. Bonner CA, Kinane MJ. Circumcision: the legal and constitutional issues. The Truth Seeker 1989 Jul/Aug;1(3):S1-S4.

Chapter 8

EDUCATING THE UNITED NATIONS ABOUT CIRCUMCISION

J. Steven Svoboda, JD
Attorneys for the Rights of the Child

Abstract: In August 2001, NOCIRC submitted an oral address and a written "intervention" to the United Nations' Sub-Commission for the Promotion and Protection of Human Rights, which became part of the official UN record. We provide the text of our written intervention. At this point in time, the Sub-Commission is the most favorable forum in which to seek UN recognition of male genital cutting (MGC) as a human rights violation. The UN and the Sub-Commission are to be congratulated for their progress in acknowledging the importance of MGC. Further work remains to expand on the UN's and the Sub-Commission's statements that (1) at least, under certain circumstances, MGC can constitute a human rights violation; and (2) anti-male sex discrimination violates human rights. Analysis of reports regarding MGC is provided by the Sub-Commission's Special Rapporteur on Traditional Practices Affecting the Health of Women and the Girl Child. We review the Sub-Commission's 1998 excision of male children from the Special Rapporteur's mandate, in apparent violation of both its own procedures and leading human rights documents.

Key words: Circumcision, United Nations, medical ethics

1.   INTRODUCTION

In July and August 2001, the political movement to secure the right to bodily integrity was officially represented for the first time at the 52nd annual meeting of the United Nations' (UN) Sub-Commission for the Promotion and Protection of Human Rights ("Sub-Commission"). Pursuant to the UN Roster Status of the National Organization of Circumcision

Flesh and Blood, Edited by Denniston et al.
Kluwer Academic/Plenum Publishers, New York 2004

89

Information Resource Centers (NOCIRC) and also unofficially representing Attorneys for the Rights of the Child (ARC), I participated in the three-week session held in Geneva, Switzerland. Tina Kimmel and Kenneth Drabik worked with me for a few days of the session. Our work included presenting an oral address and a written "intervention," which became part of the official UN record and, at least in theory, will be reviewed and considered by each Sub-Commissioner.[1] Already, the UN has recognized that circumcision, under certain circumstances, can constitute a human rights violation, and we were, among other things, seeking to obtain a general statement to that effect. The UN has also acknowledged that anti-male sex discrimination violates human rights.

2. THE SUB-COMMISSION IS CURRENTLY THE BEST FORUM BEFORE WHICH TO SEEK UN ACKNOWLEDGEMENT OF MGC

The Sub-Commission was selected as the appropriate United Nations agency to approach regarding male genital cutting (MGC), based in part on its unequalled openness to input from non-governmental organizations (NGO's) regarding proposed newly recognized human rights.

2.1 Overview of United Nations' Structure

Within the UN, human rights activities are pursued either by bodies created under the authority of the UN Charter ("Charter-based" bodies) or by bodies established under various human rights treaties ("treaty-based bodies"). The 1994 establishment of a High Commissioner on Human Rights emphasizes the increasing role human rights considerations are playing in the organization's functioning. The General Assembly, composed of all member nations of the UN, constitutes the highest UN body and its most representative decision-making organ. The Economic and Social Council (ECOSOC), the parent institution of the UN's various human rights bodies, is a subsidiary of the General Assembly. The Commission on Human Rights ("the Commission") and treaty-monitoring bodies like the Committee on the Rights of the Child are subsidiaries of ECOSOC. ECOSOC must approve all measures recommended by the Commission that involve an expenditure of funds or that need the General Assembly's attention. As a rule, ECOSOC approves the Commission's recommendations. At the final level of nesting, which is pertinent to our purposes, the Sub-Commission for the Promotion and Protection of Human Rights (whose original name was "Sub-Commission for the Prevention of Discrimination and the Protection of

Minorities") is the Commission's only sub-commission, created through a resolution passed by ECOSOC.[2] The Sub-Commission is comprised of twenty-six experts, elected by the Commission "with due regard to equitable geographic distribution," from a list of nominees submitted by UN member states.[3] Unlike the Commission, which is technically composed of member states, the Sub-Commission consists of individual "experts" who are not officially representing their country of origin. The Sub-Commission carries out studies and issues reports to the Commission regarding specific human rights conditions relating to its anti-discrimination and minority protection mandate. The Sub-Commission meets for three weeks in August every year.

2.2   Sub-Commission for the Promotion and Protection of Human Rights

The Sub-Commission appears to be the best entity to which to address a claim that MGC constitutes a human rights violation. As human rights expert Thomas Buergenthal has observed, the Sub-Commission "has traditionally been the UN institution most sympathetic to the cause of human rights."[4] Kathryn English and Adam Stapleton have written that the Sub-Commission is "notable for its independence and openness to NGOs."[5] Finally, David Weissbrodt (who happened to be a Sub-Commissioner as well as the Chairman of the Sub-Commission in 2001) and Penny Parker write that, "for NGOs the Sub-Commission has often been a more accessible forum for new ideas than other U.N. bodies."[6] The Sub-Commission's accessibility and relative willingness to entertain novel thinking is no doubt partly attributable to the aforementioned freedom of action enjoyed by its component experts.

The Sub-Commission has regularly entertained non-governmental organization's submissions of interventions regarding FGC.[7] Since genital cutting of females has been repeatedly recognized as a human rights violation by the UN's General Assembly,[8] and, not incidentally, by the Sub-Commission,[9] the expansion of this human rights category to encompass male as well as female genital mutilation fits squarely within the Sub-Commission's mandates to work towards the elimination of sex discrimination and toward the eradication of harmful traditional practices. The Sub-Commission is the best place to work to expand the contours of accepted human rights law in order to include MGC.

The threshold procedural prerequisite to any direct work with the Sub-Commission is locating an issue on which the presenting organization can hang its hat at the annual Sub-Commission meeting in Geneva. The 2001 provisional agenda of the Sub-Commission presented one agenda item that was clearly more promising than any other: Item 6(a) was dedicated to women and human rights, including "traditional practices affecting the health of women and the girl child."[10]

2.3   Sub-Commission has Power to Issue Resolutions and Undertake Studies

In 1999, the Sub-Commission underwent a reorganization and name change;[11] since then, it has been officially barred from adopting resolutions condemning particular countries. It should be noted, however, that this rule does not necessarily bar ingenious and determined Sub-Commission members from passing resolutions that formally do not name a specific country, yet, for all practical purposes focus exclusively on one or several specific nation state(s). Typically, in response to input from Sub-Commission members, UN member states and/or NGO's, the Sub-Commission can adopt resolutions condemning particular human rights violations. Criticisms of violations tend to be highly diplomatic.[12] Most frequent are expressions of "concern," such as the Sub-Commission expressed in requesting Mrs. Halima Embarek Warzazi of Morocco to study traditional practices harmful to the health of women and children.[13] Where deemed appropriate, however, the Sub-Commission on occasion will adopt harsher language that may use such terms as "deploring" and "especially disturbed."[14]

The Sub-Commission also possesses the authority to undertake studies of specific human rights conditions, which may include on-site investigations. Weissbrodt and Parker underscore the importance of this field of Sub-Commission endeavor, noting, "The Sub-Commission's principal work is the preparation of studies on new human rights issues and the drafting of new human rights standards."[15] In 1992, the Sub-Commission elected to limit the total number of studies undertaken annually to thirteen, also capping the total time period for studies at three years under normal circumstances.[16] One of the two requested actions in our written and oral interventions asked the Sub-Commission to conduct a study of MGC as a human rights violation. Such a development may serve as a precursor to the development of human rights standards to cover the subject of the report, in this case MGC.

2.4   Sub-Commission has Power to Create a Special Rapporteur or a Working Group or to Expand the Mandate of an Existing Special Rapporteur

The Sub-Commission is empowered to establish a working group to more fully explore issues of possible concern to it, to appoint a Special

Rapporteur to conduct investigations on specific issues, and to expand the mandate of an existing Special Rapporteur to encompass additional human rights issues. Requests in our written and oral interventions that a study of MGC be undertaken are necessary first steps.

One of our two requests for action in our written and oral interventions was that the Sub-Commission restore The Special Rapporteur's mandate to cover traditional practices affecting the health of women and children, as originally formulated, not merely women and the girl child, under the reduction of Mrs. Warzazi's mandate that was effected in 1997. This topic is discussed more fully *infra,* in Section 5.

3.   WRITTEN AND ORAL INTERVENTIONS

On 9 August 2001, I presented a written "intervention" or petition to the Sub-Commission.[17] Written statements are accepted by the Sub-Commission, as a subsidiary of ECOSOC, pursuant to ECOSOC Resolution 1296.[18] On 14 August 2001, I gave an oral address to a session of the Sub-Commission.[19]

In the interventions, we asked for two actions from the Sub-Commission: (1) the restoration of the Special Rapporteur's pre-1997 mandate, which — as discussed in more detail *infra* in Section 5 — covered traditional practices harmful to male children as well as female children (and women but not men); and (2) the undertaking by the Sub-Commission of a study of the issue of MGC as a human rights violation. These two requested actions were specifically designed to be relatively achievable goals.

Following is the text of the written intervention:

Contact:

J. Steven Svoboda, Esq.

National Organization of Circumcision Information Resource Centers (NOCIRC)

Geneva: 30 July–17 August 2001; J. Steven Svoboda

COMMISSION ON HUMAN RIGHTS

Sub-Commission on the Promotion and Protection of Human Rights

Fifty-third session

Agenda Item 6

TRADITIONAL PRACTICES AFFECTING THE HEALTH OF WOMEN
AND THE GIRL CHILD

**Written statement submitted by the National Organization of Circumcision
Information Resource Centers (NOCIRC), a non-governmental
organization on the Roster**

Male Circumcision

1. The National Organization of Circumcision Information Resource Centers
(NOCIRC) congratulates the Sub-Commission on its excellent work relating to
traditional practices affecting the health of women and the girl child. NOCIRC
notes with satisfaction the excellent reports prepared by Special Rapporteur Mrs.
Halima Embarek Warzazi regarding traditional practices affecting the health of
women and the girl child. NOCIRC commends in particular the excellent work
done by Mrs. Warzazi on the issue of female genital mutilation.

2. NOCIRC notes that Mrs. Warzazi's mandate originally encompassed
traditional practices affecting the health of women and children but that more
recently her mandate has apparently been redefined to focus exclusively on
traditional practices affecting the health of women and the girl child, thus
excluding traditional practices that may affect the health of the boy child. Male
circumcision apparently never has been studied as a human rights issue by the
Sub-Commission. In all places where female genital mutilation occurs, male
circumcision also occurs. Thus, elimination of one practice may go hand-in-hand
with elimination of the other.

3. Article 13 of the United Nations Charter, as well as Article 2 of the
International Covenant on Civil and Political Rights and Article 2 of the
Convention on the Rights of the Child bar discrimination on the basis of sex.
Article 7 of the Universal Declaration of Human Rights provides, "All are equal
before the law and are entitled without any discrimination to equal protection of
the law." Ms. Gay J. McDougall, as the Sub-Commission's Special Rapporteur
on Systematic Rape, Sexual Slavery and Slavery-like Practices During Armed
Conflict, stated:

> That international humanitarian law, insofar as it provides protection against
> rape and other sexual assaults, is applicable to men as well as women is
> beyond any doubt as the international human right not to be discriminated
> against (in this case on the basis of sex) does not allow derogation.[1]

Males may not be discriminated against in the application of human rights principles. United Nations experts have acknowledged that at least under certain circumstances male circumcision constitutes a human rights violation.[2]

4. The Parliament of Sweden recently voted decisively, 249 to 10, in favor of Law 2001:499, new legislation that regulates male circumcision and, in the preliminaries, also ordered a study to determine what effect the new law will have and whether male circumcision should be considered a human rights violation. Many Swedish Members of Parliament stated that male circumcision violates children's rights. The ten dissenters in the Swedish vote objected only because they supported total criminalization, rather than mere regulation, of non-therapeutic circumcision of male children.

5. Male circumcision has been stated to be a human rights violation by legislators, non-governmental organizations, and scholars. Germany awarded political asylum to a Turkish man based on his fear of enforced circumcision: "There may be...no doubt that a circumcision which has taken place against the will of the person affected shows...a violation of his physical and psychological integrity, which is of significance to asylum."

6. Numerous researchers have comprehensively documented the broad range of physical and psychological harm caused by male circumcision, including infant pain response, serious harm to infant neurological development and memory capability, the damage caused by memories of the procedure, the damage caused to self-esteem and body image, post-traumatic stress disorder, permanent impacts on sexuality, and death. Reports of death during initiations in the developing world have been appearing frequently in major press outlets. On August 6, for example, the *New York Times* ran a story mentioning that at least 35 boys have died already this year in South Africa, and ten percent or more of initiates are left with no penis or just disfigured stumps.

7. NOCIRC notes that male circumcision is a very pervasive practice throughout both the developed and developing worlds. An estimated 13.3 million male children and babies are forced to undergo male circumcision without medical indication each year. As a numerical frame of reference, 2 million females undergo some form of female genital mutilation annually. In the developed world, the procedure is typically carried out at infancy, while in the developing world it occurs any time between infancy and early adulthood depending on various factors.

8. The fact that a newborn baby can suffer pain has been conclusively proven. The harm that male circumcision causes to babies by the severe levels of pain has been repeatedly documented. The level of response to the pain and stress of

the procedure exceeds the response to blood sampling or injections and is not significantly reduced even by application of an anesthetic. Male circumcision harms women by impairing infant-mother bonding and breastfeeding.

9. Non-therapeutic male circumcision does not have any significant medical benefits justifying its routine performance upon a child. Every national medical association in the world that has considered the issue has refused to endorse routine male circumcision. Respected opponents of female genital mutilation have also questioned male circumcision and have pointed out analogies between the two practices and between false beliefs surrounding and justifying the perpetuation of the two practices. Recent research demonstrates that the average male circumcision in the developed world removes over 50% of all surface genital tissue and also a highly significant number of specialized neural end organs, including extremely specialized tissue, unique to that part of the body and fundamental to human sexual response. Research documents the long-term harm which many men experience as a result of male circumcision.

10. Research suggests that male circumcision causes behavioral changes and that some reported gender differences may actually be a result of male circumcision.

11. Complications in the developed world occur with a frequency of between 2-5% or more depending on the definition applied. A significant number of deaths occur each year. One study of male circumcision in the developing world found that 9% of the boys died, 52% lost all or most of their penile shaft skin, 14% developed severe infectious lesions, 10% lost their glans penis, and 5% lost their entire penis. This represents only those boys who completed travel to the hospital. The true complication rate is likely to be higher.

12. While supporting Mrs. Warzazi's admirable work on traditional practices specifically affecting women and the girl-child, NOCIRC respectfully requests that the Sub-Commission also focus attention on traditional practices that specifically affect the male child, such as male circumcision. NOCIRC notes that the International Covenant on Civil and Political Rights, the Convention on the Rights of the Child, and other relevant treaties are applicable both to males and females, and that discrimination against either gender in their application is forbidden.

13. Legislation or human rights provisions that protect against female genital mutilation and not male circumcision violate the human rights of the boy child. Ample evidence proves the serious harm caused by male circumcision. Logically, any difference in severity between female genital mutilation and male circumcision, even if proven, does not justify the neglect of the latter practice.

14. Any alteration of children's genitals performed without absolute medical indication violates human rights. Male circumcision violates the International Covenant on Civil and Political Rights, the International Covenant on Economic, Social and Cultural Rights, the Convention on the Rights of the Child, and other documents. Relevant rights include the rights to security of the person, to the highest attainable standard of health, and to protection from "all forms of physical or mental violence, injury or abuse, neglect or negligent treatment, maltreatment or exploitation, including sexual abuse." Article 24.3 of the Convention on the Rights of the Child calls on states to "take all effective and appropriate measures with a view to abolishing traditional practices prejudicial to the health of children," terminology that — as human rights scholars such as Jacqueline Smith have commented — is fully applicable to male circumcision.

Conclusions

15. Male circumcision causes permanent and severe harm and violates human rights.

16. NOCIRC asks that the mandate of the Special Rapporteur on Traditional Practices Affecting the Health of Women and the Girl Child be revised to again encompass traditional practices affecting the health of women and children.

17. NOCIRC asks that the Sub-Commission undertake a study of male circumcision as a human rights violation.

Notes

1. Contemporary forms of slavery: systematic rape, sexual slavery and slavery-like practices during armed conflict: final report submitted by Ms. Gay J. McDougall, Special Rapporteur (E/CN.4/Sub.2/1998/13, para. 24).

2. United Nations Security Council. Commission of Experts' Final Report [on the Former Yugoslavia] (S/1994/674, part IV, section F).

4.   RECOGNITION OF MGC

Numerous eminent scholars such as Jacqueline Smith[20] and Margaret Somerville[21] have noted the legal and human rights problems implicated by MGC. Moreover, the Sub-Commission and other UN bodies have already repeatedly acknowledged MGC's status as a potential human rights violation as well as males' human right to equal protection against sex discrimination.

Sub-Commissioner Ms. Gay J. McDougall, the Sub-Commission's expert on systematic rape and sexual slavery, advised the Sub-Commission that sex discrimination against males violates international law.[22] Ms. McDougall stressed that human rights must protect both males and females from all forms of sexual assault. Several documents released by the United Nations recognize various forms of sexual assault on males, including circumcision, as torture and as a human rights violation.[23] Since 1999, the Committee on the Rights of the Child has placed its concerns about male circumcision on record no fewer than three separate times. In 1999, the Committee called on South Africa to "please provide additional information on the traditional practice of male circumcision and outline the programs undertaken and/or envisaged to eliminate this practice and promote awareness of its harmful effects on boys."[24] In 2000, the Committee expressed its concern that, in South Africa, male circumcision is in some instances carried out in unsafe medical conditions. The Committee also recommended that South Africa "take effective measures, including training for practitioners and awareness-raising, to ensure the health of boys and protect against unsafe medical conditions during the practice of male circumcision."[25] Finally, in 2001, the Committee expressed its concerns with health risks linked to male circumcision in Lesotho.[26]

Male circumcision is specifically cited as a sexual assault to which men have been subjected in the final report of the UN commission of experts assembled to report on humanitarian law violations in the former Yugoslavia.[27] The Fourth Report on War Crimes in the Former Yugoslavia (Part II) reports as "torture of prisoners" circumcisions performed on Bosnian Serb soldiers by Muslim and Mujahedin troops.[28] The Final Report notes that, where such acts of mutilation constitute "serious international violations directed against the protected persons, in contradistinction to a fate befalling them merely as a side-effect," they are prohibited by common article 3 of the four Geneva Conventions of 1949 and by Protocol II to the Geneva Conventions. Clearly, recognition of the human rights problems posed by male circumcision is developing in the United Nations.

5.   THE SUB-COMMISSION'S APPARENTLY IMPROPER REDEFINITION OF THE SPECIAL RAPPORTEUR'S MANDATE

The Sub-Commission is due sincere congratulations for its hard work to date, acknowledging the importance of MGC as a human rights violation. At the same time, the Sub-Commission appears to have violated its own procedures as well as some central UN documents through its 1997 redefinition of the mandate of the Special Rapporteur on Traditional

Practices, which excluded male children (along with the previously excluded male adults). Such unequal treatment based on sex clearly and gravely violates core human rights principles, including Article 7 of the Universal Declaration of Human Rights, which states: "All are equal before the law and are entitled without any discrimination to equal protection of the law. All are entitled to equal protection against any discrimination in violation of the Declaration and against any incitement to such discrimination." Article 2 of the Universal Declaration, which provides, "Everyone is entitled to all the rights and freedoms set forth in this Declaration, without distinction of any kind, such as... sex..." The Sub-Commission's action also directly contravenes Article 2 of the Convention on the Rights of the Child, which demands that the rights of each child be ensured without discrimination based on sex or other listed factors. Such policies also violate Article 1, paragraph 3 of the Charter of the United Nations, which includes among the purposes of the United Nations promoting and encouraging respect for human rights and fundamental freedoms for all without distinction as to race, sex, language, or religion, as well as Charter Article 55(c), which states that the UN "shall promote... universal respect for, and observance of, human rights and fundamental freedoms for all without distinction as to race, sex, language, or religion."[29] All members and all subdivisions of the United Nations are bound by all Charter provisions. Therefore, a human rights violation occurs where males are discriminated against by not enjoying the UN's enforcement of their right to protection from genital mutilation. Moreover, the Sub-Commission's actions violate its own findings, which, as discussed in Section 4, *infra*, affirm that MGC is a human rights violation and that discrimination against males violates human rights.[30]

5.1   Historical Development of the Special Rapporteur

The Special Rapporteur's position was first created at a 1985 meeting of the Sub-Commission's Working Group on Slavery. For the following twelve years, the Special Rapporteur's efforts on traditional practices principally addressed issues directly relevant only to girls (FGC, honor killings, early marriage, son preference, infanticide and neglect of girls, "crimes of honor," etc.) while secondarily working on some issues affecting both male and female children (harmful traditional healing practices, harmful childbirth practices, etc.). In 1997, in an apparent violation of the Sub-Commission's normal procedure as well as the requirements of core UN documents, the Special Rapporteur's mandate was silently reduced during the Sub-Commission's 49th session in July-August 1997. As late as 25 June 1997, one Sub-Commission document still refers to the "Special Rapporteur on traditional practices affecting the health of women and children."[31] But by the time the Sub-Commission meeting was nearing its conclusion and it issued its report on the session, Mrs. Warzazi's mandate had been changed to cover "traditional practices affecting the health of women and the girl child."[32] Evidently no substantive discussion of this seemingly highly significant change ever occurred, nor was the change of title ever alluded to in any Sub-Commission document. Seven years ago, the Commission may have signaled the Sub-Commission regarding its greater interest in FGC relative to MGC. The Commission directed two paragraphs in its 1996 resolution on the rights of the child to the alleged need for "paying particular attention to the obstacles faced by the girl child" and encouraging states "to enact and enforce legislation" addressing, *inter alia*, FGC.[33] It said nothing regarding MGC.

Although the Sub-Commission evidently does not have a rule speaking directly to this issue, the UN as a whole as well as its constituent parts, including the Sub-Commission, are institutions that above all value protocol and established procedure. It is highly irregular for the mandate and title of any officer of the Sub-Commission to be altered without discussion or even official notice, particularly a position as influential as the Special Rapporteur on Traditional Practices. I scanned numerous documents from Sub-Commission history and reviewed all relevant procedures[34-35] without being able to locate any viable procedure on which the Sub-Commission could claim to rely in taking this evidently unprecedented step.

5.2   Analysis of the Special Rapporteur's Work Regarding MGC

The Special Rapporteur deserves praise for her sustained commitment to publicizing and rooting out FGC. However, her actions unfortunately demonstrate differential treatment of MGC and FGC despite her acknowledged receipt of numerous communications regarding MGC. For example, in January of 1997, the Special Rapporteur received a questionnaire about male and female circumcision, to which she replied by inaccurately suggesting that "the circumcision of male children did not concern the United Nations as only female circumcision was deemed a harmful practice to be eradicated. Consequently, it would seem inappropriate to consider under one head both female circumcision which is harmful to health and male circumcision which has no undesirable effect and it [sic] even considered to be beneficial."[36] The Special Rapporteur provides no support for her assertions.

In a report issued in 2000, the Special Rapporteur mentions in one paragraph receiving mail concerning male circumcision[37] and later writes:

For the sake of transparency, the Special Rapporteur would like to mention the fact that she has received a few letters condemning male circumcision. In order to close once and for all an acrimonious debate, which has led to personal attacks against herself, she would like to recall that her mandate by the Sub-Commission on the Promotion and Protection of Human Rights concerns traditional practices affecting the health of women and the girl child. The same mandate applies with regard to the General Assembly or other United Nations bodies. By restricting herself to female circumcision, the Special Rapporteur is therefore only keeping to her terms of reference. Furthermore, she considers that the harmful effects of male circumcision cannot in any way be compared or equated with the violence, danger and risk faced by girl children and women.[38] [emphasis in original]

A number of distortions of the truth are evident here. The Special Rapporteur's references to the coverage of her mandate and her suggestion that she is "only keeping to her terms of reference" are literally correct but highly misleading. It is true that, *since August 1997*, her mandate covered only women and the girl child. At the time the Special Rapporteur made this comment, her time with a mandate covering only girls represented less than three years of a total of 15 years working on the topic. She fails to allude to the preceding 12 years, during which her mandate also covered male children. Similarly, her suggestion that "the same mandate" applies to the General Assembly or other UN bodies, while technically correct, is again highly misleading. The Special Rapporteur implies that other UN bodies have also elected to concentrate on traditional practices affecting women and the girl child, whereas the truth is other UN bodies' actions on the topic occur as reactions to the reports and actions of the Sub-Commission and its Special Rapporteur. A comprehensive search of UN documents issued since the mid-1990s by both charter-based and treaty-based entities on the topic of traditional practices harmful to women and the girl child disclosed only Sub-Commission documents and documents issued by the General Assembly,[39-40] ECOSOC,[41] the Commission,[42] and the Committee on the Rights of the Child,[43-44] all in response to actions or reports instigated by the Special Rapporteur. Next, the Special Rapporteur makes a statement regarding the alleged non-comparability of the harmful effects of male and female circumcision that can only be considered a *non sequitur*. No citation is provided and of course this begs the question: Even if it is true that the harm of MGC, which even the Special Rapporteur concedes does exist, is greatly exceeded in magnitude by the harm caused by FGC, this does not justify the UN and the Special Rapporteur failing to act to correct human rights violated by MGC. Human rights protections are not subject to being competitively balanced against each other in the scales of international justice to determine which should be enforced.[45]

The 2000 document contains further misleading claims in the following paragraph. Mrs. Warzazi writes:

> To close this aside, the Special Rapporteur might draw attention to a study published at the beginning of the year by the University of Washington (Seattle), which concludes that the great majority of boys suffer no complications as a result of circumcision. What is more, the Sunday Times (United Kingdom) of 26 March 2000 published a scientific study carried out by specialists of Melbourne University in Australia, according to which male circumcision may be related to a lower risk of HIV transmission from women to men.[46]

Setting aside the imprecise suggestion that the *Sunday Times* published a scientific study rather than a news story regarding such a study, it can easily be shown that both articles referenced by Warzazi are flawed and unworthy of UN citation. As Dennis Harrison adroitly noted, the first one, by Christakis, et al.,[47] "appears to confirm that a medically unnecessary surgical intervention is being undertaken in an ethical vacuum on the basis of limited scientific understanding."[48] After reporting that certain complications occur twenty times more frequently in circumcised infants than in intact males, the authors somehow manage to conclude that circumcision remains a "relatively safe procedure."[49] They also fail to address the important ethical, legal, and human rights issues raised when a medically unnecessary surgical operation is carried out on a person who cannot speak for himself.

The second article the Special Rapporteur mentions, by Short and Szabo,[50] is similarly fallacious. This notoriously flawed article provoked a torrent of letters responding to and debunking its claims.[51] As Robert S. Van Howe has pointed out, the authors' simple-minded tallying of studies without allowing for confounding factors is "both unscientific and misleading."[52] The futility of Short and Szabo's attempt to blame male genital integrity for HIV is clear, since the United States has both the highest circumcision rate in the developed world, estimated at seventy-seven percent,[53] and the highest incidence of sexually transmitted disease infection amongst the same nations.[54] Systematic review, using meta-analysis of studies regarding circumcision status and HIV, has shown a substantial degree of heterogeneity across studies,[55] naturally casting serious doubt on the validity of superficial summary surveys such as that of Short and Szabo. Because many diverse considerations affect sexual behavior and vulnerability to HIV, blaming it on normal anatomy is bad science and an even worse human rights policy. The numerous distortions and mistakes of fact found in these few sentences were presumably not inadvertent errors, since the entire first paragraph appears again almost *verbatim* in another report made in 2001, including a concession — again repeated in two separate paragraphs — that she continues to receive mail relating to male circumcision.[56] Interestingly, in the more recent document, the Special

Rapporteur backs off from alluding to "personal attacks" and deletes the two medical references on which she relies in the previous report.

In short, the Special Rapporteur's work on MGC suffers from superficiality regarding even relatively basic medical and human rights aspects of the procedure, flaws not evident in her efforts to halt female genital cutting.

5.3   Bringing the Mandate into Compliance

Thus, the Sub-Commission finds itself violating the UN's own human rights standards. The requested reinstitution of the Special Rapporteur's mandate to encompass traditional practices harming male children would promote compliance with equal protection and non-discrimination requirements applicable under both human rights principles and the national laws of numerous countries.[57] The requested change would be invaluable in promoting universal genital integrity and would remind the Special Rapporteur regarding the need to use her office's resources to address both FGC and MGC.

6.   CONCLUSION

The United Nations and its Sub-Commission for the Promotion and Protection of Human Rights have made an admirable start in recognizing MGC as a human rights violation under certain circumstances and, by accepting into their official records, an intervention documenting that male genital cutting contravenes human rights principles. The UN and the Sub-Commission deserve further praise for acknowledging that sex discrimination against males constitutes a human rights violation. Nevertheless, further work remains to be done. The Sub-Commission's unacknowledged reduction of the Special Rapporteur's mandate contravenes UN principles on both substantive and procedural grounds and should be reversed immediately. We are confident that the UN and the Sub-Commission will continually expand upon their already laudable recognition that male circumcision is an issue that must be addressed in the name of humanity.

REFERENCES

1. *See* Rodley N. United Nations non-treaty procedures for dealing with human rights violations. In: Hannum H, editor. Guide to International Human Rights Practice (2nd ed.) Philadelphia: University of Pennsylvania Press;1992. p. 60-85 [here, p. 78-79.]

2. United Nations Economic and Social Council. Resolution 9(II) (21 June 1946).
3. United Nations High Commissioner for Human Rights, United Nations Sub-Commission on Prevention of Discrimination and Protection of Minorities. United Nations Human Rights Website; 1996-2001. [cited 27 February 2002].
   URL: http://www.unhchr.ch/html/menu2/2/sc.htm.
4. Buergenthal T. International human rights in a nutshell. St. Paul, MN: West Publishing Co.;1995. p. 83.
5. English K, Stapleton S. The Human rights handbook. Kenwyn, South Africa: Juta & Co.;1997. p. 9.
6. Weissbrodt D, Parker P. The U.N. Commission on Human Rights, its Sub-Commission, and related procedures: an orientation manual. Minneapolis: Minnesota Advocates for Human Rights;1993. p.3.
7. *See, e.g.,* United Nations Commission on Human Rights, Sub-Commission on Prevention of Discrimination and Protection of Minorities, forty-sixth session, agenda item 4. Review of further developments with which the Sub-Commission has been concerned--written statement submitted by the International Association of Educators for World Peace, a non-governmental organization on the Roster. UN Doc. No. ECN.4/Sub.2/1994/NGO/36 (1994).
8. *See, e.g.,* United Nations General Assembly Resolution 52/99 (1997).
9. *See, e.g.,* United Nations Sub-Commission on Prevention of Discrimination and Protection of Minorities. Follow-up report of the special rapporteur on traditional practices affecting the health of women and children, Mrs. Halima Embarek Warzizi, UN Doc. No. E/CN.4/Sub.2/1997/10 and Add.1 (1997).
10. United Nations High Commissioner for Human Rights, United Nations Sub-Commission on Prevention of Discrimination and Protection of Minorities. Agenda. United Nations Human Rights Website; 1996-2001. [cited, 27 Feb 2002].
    http://www.unhchr.ch/huridocda/huridoca.nsf/(Symbol)/E.CN.4.Sub.2.2001.1.Rev.1.En?O pendocument. UN Doc. No. E/CN.4/Sub.2/2001/Rev.1 (15 May 2001).
11. United Nations High Commissioner for Human Rights, United Nations Sub-Commission on Prevention of Discrimination and Protection of Minorities. United Nations Human Rights Website; 1996-2001. [cited 27 February 2002].
    URL: http://www.unhchr.ch/html/menu2/2/sc.htm.
12. Brennan K. The influence of cultural relativism on international human rights law: female circumcision as a case study. Law and Inequality 1989;7:367-398. [here, p. 394 and note 132.]
13. United Nations Commission on Human Rights, Sub-Commission on Prevention of Discrimination and Protection of Minorities. Resolution 1988/34, UN Doc. No. E/CN.4/Sub.2/1988/45 (1988), para. 62.
14. United Nations Commission on Human Rights, Sub-Commission on Prevention of Discrimination and Protection of Minorities. Report of the Sub-Commission on Prevention of Discrimination and Protection of Minorities on its 37th session, Geneva, 6-31 August 1984. UN Doc. No. E/CN.4/Sub. 2/1984/43 (19 October 1984), p. 1.
15. Weissbrodt D, Parker P. The U.N. Commission on Human Rights, its Sub-Commission, and related procedures: an orientation manual. Minneapolis: Minnesota Advocates for Human Rights;1993. p.19.
16. United Nations Commission on Human Rights, Sub-Commission on the Promotion and Protection of Human Rights. Guidelines for the application by the Sub-Commission on the Promotion and Protection of Human Rights of the rules of procedure of the functional commissions of the Economic and Social Council and other decisions and practices

relating thereto. Sub-Commission Resolution 1999/114, annex. UN Doc. No.HR/NONE/2001/126, para. 27-8 [Guideline 1.]

17. Attorneys for the Rights of the Child. Report of the Sub-Commission on the Promotion and Protection of Human Rights on its fifty-third session--written statement submitted by the National Organization of Circumcision Information Resource Centers (NOCIRC), a non-governmental organization on the Roster--male circumcision;9 August 2001. [cited 6 March 2002]. UN Doc. No. E/CN.4/Sub.2/2002/NGO/1 (23 March 2002).

18. United Nations Economic and Social Council, forty-fourth session. Economic and Social Council resolution 1296 (XLIV) on consultative arrangements (23 May 1968), para. 23-24.

19. Attorneys for the Rights of the Child. Report of the Sub-Commission on the Promotion and Protection of Human Rights on its fifty-third session--written statement submitted by the National Organization of Circumcision Information Resource Centers (NOCIRC), a non-governmental organization on the Roster--male circumcision; 9 August 2001. [cited 6 March 2002]. UN Doc. No. E/CN.4/Sub.2/2002/NGO/1 (23 March 2002).

20. Smith J. Male circumcision and the rights of the child. In: Bulterman M, Hendriks A, Smith J, editors. To Baehr in Our Minds: Essays in Human Rights from the Heart of the Netherlands (SIM Special No. 21). Utrecht, Netherlands: Netherlands Institute of Human Rights (SIM), University of Utrecht;1998. p. 465-498.

21. Somerville MA. Altering baby boys' bodies: the ethics of infant male circumcision. In: Somerville MA. The ethical canary: science, society and the human spirit. Toronto:Viking;2000.

22. United Nations Commission on Human Rights, Sub-Commission on Prevention of Discrimination and Protection of Minorities. Contemporary forms of slavery: systematic rape, sexual slavery and slavery-like practices during armed conflict: final report submitted by Ms. Gay J. McDougall, Special Rapporteur. UN Doc. No. E/CN.4/Sub.2/1998/13 (22 June 1998), para. 24.

23. Amnesty International Bermuda. Bodily integrity for both: the obligation of Amnesty International to recognize all forms of genital mutilation of males as human rights violations. Hamilton, Bermuda: Amnesty International Bermuda;1998. p. 15.

24. United Nations Committee on the Rights of the Child, twenty-third session. Implementation of the Convention on the Rights of the Child; 1996-2001. [cited 6 March 2002].
http://www.unhchr.ch/tbs/doc.nsf/385c2add1632f4a8c12565a9004dc311/30d2b78b71b39 92a8025682d005ae379?OpenDocument.
UN Doc. No. CRC/C/Q/ SAFR/1 (13-17 September 1999), para. 21.

25. United Nations Committee on the Rights of the Child, twenty-third session. Concluding observations of the Committee on the Rights of the Child: South Africa; 1996-2001. [cited 27 February 2002].URL:
http://www.unhchr.ch/tbs/doc.nsf/385c2add1632f4a8c12565a9004dc311/6e861f881eca1b 1e8025687f005a805b?OpenDocument&Highlight=0,CRC%2FC%2F15%2FAdd.122.
UN Doc. No. CRC/C/15/Add.122 (23 February 2000), para. 33.

26. United Nations Committee on the Rights of the Child, twenty-sixth session. Concluding observations of the Committee on the Rights of the Child: Lesotho; 1996-2001. [cited 27 February 2002].
http://www.unhchr.ch/tbs/doc.nsf/385c2add1632f4a8c12565a9004dc311/ae3810fc637a1d 6ec12569ee0032b0a3?OpenDocument. UN Doc No. CRC/C/15/Add. 147 (February 2001), para. 43.

27. United Nations Commission of Experts' Final Report; 1996-2001. [cited 27 February 2002]. URL: http://uwe.ac.uk/facults/ess/comexpert/I-II.htm. UN Doc. No. S/1994/674 (1994), section IV.F

28. United Nations. Fourth Report on War Crimes in the Former Yugoslavia (Part II): Torture of Prisoners, 3 March 2002; 1996-2001. [cited 27 February 2002].
URL: http://www.haverford.edu/relg/sells/reports/4thB.html.

29. Charter of the United Nations, 26 June 1945.

30. United Nations Commission on Human Rights, Sub-Commission on Prevention of Discrimination and Protection of Minorities. Contemporary forms of slavery: systematic rape, sexual slavery and slavery-like practices during armed conflict: final report submitted by Ms. Gay J. McDougall, Special Rapporteur. UN Doc. No. E/CN.4/Sub.2/1998/13 (22 June 1998), para. 24.

31. United Nations Commission on Human Rights, Sub-Commission on Prevention of Discrimination and Protection of Minorities, forty-ninth session, provisional agenda item 5(a). The implementation of the human rights of women—traditional practices affecting the health of women and children--Follow-up report of the Special Rapporteur on traditional practices affecting the health of women and children, Mrs. Halima Embarek Warzazi. UN Doc. No. E/CN.4/Sub.2/1997/10 (25 June 1997).

32. United Nations Commission on Human Rights, Sub-Commission on Prevention of Discrimination and Protection of Minorities, forty-ninth session. Report of the Sub-Commission on Prevention of Discrimination and Protection of Minorities on its forty-ninth session. UN Doc. No. E/CN.4/1998/2, E/CN.4/Sub.2/1997/50 (29 August 1997).

33. United Nations Commission on Human Rights. Rights of the Child. Commission on Human Rights resolution 1996/85. UN Doc. No. E/CN.4/RES/1996/85 (24 April 1996), paras. 44-45.

34. *See* United Nations Commission on Human Rights, Sub-Commission on the Promotion and Protection of Human Rights. Guidelines for the application by the Sub-Commission on the Promotion and Protection of Human Rights of the rules of procedure of the functional commissions of the Economic and Social Council and other decisions and practices relating thereto. Sub-Commission Resolution 1999/114, annex. UN Doc. No.HR/NONE/2001/126, paras. 27-8.

35. *See also* United Nations High Commissioner for Human Rights. Rules of procedure of the functional commissions of the Economic and Social Council. United Nations Human Rights Website; 1996-2001. [cited 27 February 2002].
URL: http://www.unhchr.ch/html/menu2/2/rules.htm

36. United Nations Commission on Human Rights, Sub-Commission on Prevention of Discrimination and Protection of Minorities. The implementation of the human rights of women—traditional practices affecting the health of women and children; 1996-2001. [cited 27 February 2002].
http://www.unhchr.ch/Huridocda/Huridoca.nsf/TestFrame/c6e77e47e54b2dab8025665d00 526549?Opendocument. UN Doc. No. E/CN.4/Sub.2/1997/10 (25 June 1997), para. 18.

37. Protection of Human Rights. Other issues—traditional practices affecting the health of women and the girl child—fifth report on the situation regarding the elimination of traditional practices affecting the health of women and the girl child, produced by Mrs. Halima Embarek Warzazi pursuant to Sub-Commission resolution 2000/10;[cited 4 July 2001]. URL:
http://www.unhchr.ch/Huridocda/Huridoca.nsf/TestFrame/156783fc6d8426d6c1256aa900 300cd3?Opendocument, para. 49.

38. United Nations Commission on Human Rights, Sub-Commission for the Promotion and Protection of Human Rights. Other issues—traditional practices affecting the health of

women and the girl child—fifth report on the situation regarding the elimination of traditional practices affecting the health of women and the girl child, produced by Mrs. Halima Embarek Warzazi pursuant to Sub-Commission resolution 2000/10;[cited 4 July 2001]. URL: http://www.unhchr.ch/Huridocda/Huridoca.nsf/TestFrame/156783fc6d8426d6c1256aa900 300cd3?Opendocument, para. 54.

39. United Nations General Assembly. Advancement of women—report of the Third Committee; 1996-2001. [cited 27 February 2002]. http://www.unhchr.ch/Huridocda/Huridoca.nsf/TestFrame/e7bca0a35b1786258025684600 387d25?Opendocument. UN Doc. No. A/54/598 (23 November 1999), sec. III.

40. United Nations General Assembly Resolution 55/66, 31 January 2001.

41. United Nations Economic and Social Council. Report of the Economic and Social Council for 2001; 1996-2001. [cited 27 February 2002]. http://www.unhchr.ch/huridocda/huridoca.nsf/AllSymbols/9A06461FF17CFA86C1256AF 800583E8E/$File/N0155285.doc?OpenElement. UN Doc. No. A/56/3 (26 September 2001), p. 73, para. 247.

42. *See, e.g.,* United Nations Economic and Social Council. Report on the fifty-sixth session—supplement no. 3; 1996-2001. [cited 27 February 2002]. http://www.unhchr.ch/Huridocda/Huridoca.nsf/0/171a288fca4bb1c8c125697d0046b5c0/$ FILE/G0014048.doc. UN Doc. No. E/2000/23, E/CN.4/2000/167 (20 March-28 April 2000), p. 200, 336-7.

43. United Nations Committee on the Rights of the Child, nineteenth session. Implementation of the Convention on the Rights of the Child; 1996-2001. [cited 27 February 2002]. http://www.unhchr.ch/tbs/doc.nsf/385c2add1632f4a8c12565a9004dc311/c9808f27371771 388025668e0032b31b?OpenDocument. UN Doc. No. CRC/C/SR.478 (23 September 1998), para. 7.

44. United Nations Committee on the Rights of the Child, nineteenth session. Implementation of the Convention on the Rights of the Child; 1996-2001. [cited 27 February 2002]. http://www.unhchr.ch/tbs/doc.nsf/385c2add1632f4a8c12565a9004dc311/8eb6429fdd7c2c 5680256804004c5f7b?OpenDocument. UN Doc. No. CRC/C/SR.558 (1 October 1999), para. 8.

45. Svoboda JS. Routine infant male circumcision: examining the human rights and constitutional issues. In: Denniston GC, Milos MF, editors. Sexual mutilations: a human tragedy. New York: Plenum Press;1997:205-15. [here, p. 213.]

46. United Nations Commission on Human Rights, Sub-Commission for the Promotion and Protection of Human Rights. Other issues—traditional practices affecting the health of women and the girl child—fifth report on the situation regarding the elimination of traditional practices affecting the health of women and the girl child, produced by Mrs. Halima Embarek Warzazi pursuant to Sub-Commission resolution 2000/10. [cited 4 July 2001]. http://www.unhchr.ch/Huridocda/Huridoca.nsf/TestFrame/156783fc6d8426d6c1256aa900 300cd3?Opendocument, para. 55.

47. Christakis DA, Harvey E, Zerr DM, Feudtner C, Wright JA, Connell FA. A trade-off analysis of routine newborn circumcision. Pediatrics 2000;105(1):Suppl 1:246-9.

48. Harrison D. A trade-off analysis of routine newborn circumcision. Pediatrics 2000;106(4):954.

49. Christakis DA, Harvey E, Zerr DM, Feudtner C, Wright JA, Connell FA. A trade-off analysis of routine newborn circumcision. Pediatrics 2000;105(1):Suppl 1:246-9. [here, p. 248.]

50. Szabo R, Short RV. How does male circumcision protect against HIV infection? BMJ 2000;320:1592-4.

51. *See, e.g.,* Dalton J. BXO does not require treatment by circumcision. British Medical Journal, 1 October 2000. [cited 23 November 2002]. URL: bmj.com/cgi/eletters/321/7264/792#10014; Hill G. Circumcision of male children may vanish from British medical practice. British Medical Journal, 4 October 2000. [cited 23 November 2002]. URL: bmj.com/cgi/eletters/321/7264/780#10085; Barichello L. Infant circumcision not warranted by study. British Medical Journal, 11 October 2000. [cited 23 November 2002]. URL: bmj.com/cgi/eletters/320/7249/1592#8294; Boyle G. Circumcision of children: criminal assault. British Medical Journal, 11 October 2000. [cited 23 November 2002]. URL: bmj.com/cgi/eletters/320/7249/1592#8297; Shale T. Circumcision: not the way to prevent AIDS. British Medical Journal, 12 October 2000. [cited 23 November 2002]. URL: bmj.com/cgi/eletters/320/7249/1592#8315; Gustavson EL. Circumcision complication rate. British Medical Journal, 13 October 2000. [cited 23 November 2002]. URL: bmj.com/cgi/eletters/320/7249/1592#8331.

52. Van Howe RS. A little bit of science wouldn't have gone amiss. British Medical Journal; 19 July 2000. [cited 6 March 2002].
URL: http://bmj.com/cgi/eletters/320/7249/1592#8260.

53. Laumann, EO, Masi CM, Zuckerman EW. Circumcision in the United States. *JAMA* 1997;277(13):1052-1057.

54. World Health Organization. The current global situation of the HIV/AIDS pandemic. Geneva: World Health Organization; 3 July 1995.

55. *See* de Vincenzi I, Mertens T. Male circumcision: a role in HIV prevention? AIDS 1994;8(2):153-160.

56. United Nations Commission on Human Rights, Sub-Commission on Prevention of Discrimination and Protection of Minorities. The implementation of the human rights of women—traditional practices affecting the health of women and the girl child—fourth report on the situation regarding the elimination of traditional practices affecting the health of women and the girl child, produced by Mrs. Halima Embarek Warzazi pursuant to Sub-Commission resolution 1999/13; 1996-2001. [cited 27 February 2002]. URL: http://www.unhchr.ch/Huridocda/Huridoca.nsf/TestFrame/c6e77e47e54b2dab8025665d00 526549?Opendocument. UN Doc. No. E/CN.4/Sub.2/1997/10 (25 June 1997), paras. 77, 82.

57. *See, e.g.,* United States Constitution, Amendments V and XIV.

Chapter 9

CIRCUMCISION OF BOYS

Time for Doctors to Reconsider

Yngve Hofvander, MD
Professor, Uppsala University, Sweden; Former Head International Child Health

Abstract: This paper provides an in-depth analysis of the current legal and medical status of male circumcision within the ethical framework of the United Nations Convention on the Rights of the Child.

Key words: Circumcision, United Nations, medical ethics

1.   INTRODUCTION

The United Nations Convention on the Rights of the Child, from 1989, states, in Article 19, that States "shall take all appropriate legislative, administrative, social, and educational measures to protect the child from all forms of physical or mental violation, injury or abuse..." Article 24.3 urges all States "to take all effective and appropriate measures with a view to abolishing traditional practices prejudicial to the health of children." Article 37 states that: "No child shall be subjected to torture or other cruel, inhuman or degrading treatment . . . ."

In the *UNICEF Implementation Handbook for the Convention* (1998), it states in relation to Article 24.3 that a review is to be undertaken regarding "all forms of genital mutilation and circumcision." Other traditional practices to be reviewed include "binding, scarring, burning, branding, forced holding under water" and similar cruel treatment of children.

Male circumcision is often — in analogy with the circumcision of girls — referred to as male genital mutilation (MGM) because it results in the removal and destruction of part of an organ that has highly specialized functions. This term will be used here along with circumcision.

Flesh and Blood, Edited by Denniston et al.
Kluwer Academic/Plenum Publishers, New York 2004

109

Male circumcision is performed on a large scale in the following four population groups. The figures are approximate, being based on fertility rates in the respective population groups (*UNICEF: State of the World's Children, 2002*), and based on a conservative estimate of a circumcision rate of eighty percent (except for the United States where the circumcision rate can be documented with greater accuracy).

Table 1. Worldwide Circumcision Rates

Motivation	Target Group	Number Circumcised Per Year
Religious	Jews	100,000
Religious	Muslims	12 million
Tribal ritual	Sub Saharan Africa	9 million
Medical ritualism	United States	1.2 million

While the literature on neonatal circumcision in the United States is abundant, it is remarkable how little is known and reported about the circumcision practices among the other groups listed above, even though circumcision is the most frequently performed surgery in these cultures.

2.   BACKGROUND

It is impossible to determine why circumcision was first introduced, whether it was first practiced as a partial and symbolic act of castration, a ritualized act of degradation and humiliation, a cultic blood rite done for superstitious reasons, a bizarre fertility ritual, or simply a ritual phenomenon intended to stigmatize the victim as a member of a particular ethnic group.

The first historical evidence for the practice of circumcision dates to Old Kingdom Egypt (2649-2134 BC). The sixth-dynasty (2349-2134 BC) funerary relief found at the Mastaba of Ankhmahor in the cemetery at Saqqara seems to depict a form of penile mutilation (possibly a dorsal slit rather than a full circumcision) being imposed on an adult. The operation was not universally imposed, but was limited to certain members of the priestly caste and to slaves.[1] Classic Greek sources claimed that the practice spread from this region of Northern Africa to other Near and Middle Eastern tribes.[2]

According to Israelite legend recorded in the priestly (ca. 950 BC) revision of the Old Testament book of Genesis 1:17, Abraham, the mythical progenitor of the Hebrews, received a revelation from the god Jehovah instructing him to enter into a covenant with him. The provision was that the ninety-nine-year-old Abraham should circumcise himself along with all the other male members of his household as well as his slaves. In exchange, he would see his progeny increase and have dominion over the land of Israel. Due to the pervasiveness of this myth, infant male circumcision evolved into one of the most tenacious blood rituals among the Jews. In recent years, however, the custom is more often reinterpreted as an ethnic marker than a cultic sacrifice to a supernatural deity and is much less rigidly observed.[3]

The history of circumcision among Muslims is especially perplexing because circumcision is nowhere mentioned in the Koran and is therefore an inauthentic Islamic religious ritual.[4] In commentaries on the Koran, first written down hundreds of years after the time of Mohamed, apocryphal statements are made from which it may be possible to conclude that both male and female Muslims should be circumcised. As among Jews, Muslim circumcision serves more as an ethnic marker than a genuinely religious ritual.

The origin and purpose of male circumcision in sub-Saharan Africa is lost in a historical mist. The medical literature dealing with tribal African circumcision is indeed scanty, except for occasional articles focusing on complications, especially those occurring in South Africa. Among some tribal groups, the operation is performed prior to puberty as an initiation rite, graphically marking the boy as having attained the status of adulthood. In urban areas of Africa, the operation may be performed earlier in imitation of American medical rituals. Here again, in the African context where tribal divisions are taken very seriously, circumcision among those sub-Saharan groups that practice it is a deeply rooted tradition that emphatically serves as an ethnic marker.

In the United States, the medical profession introduced male circumcision about 150 years ago as prophylaxis, punishment, and treatment for masturbation.[5] Soon, doctors augmented the incredibly long list of serious diseases that circumcision was supposed to cure or prevent to include such conditions as epilepsy, idiocy, asthma, tuberculosis, rheumatism, and spinal paralysis.[6] Circumcision was made into a quasi-compulsory neonatal surgical procedure after the Second World War for medical-sounding reasons whose authenticity is similarly dubious.

3.   THE FORESKIN

Up to the seventh fetal week, the male and the female genitals are identical. Thereafter, male hormones initiate the development of male genitals. In the twelfth week, the prepuce is formed as a double pleat of skin that grows down to cover the glans. The inner layer of the prepuce and the glans remain attached until about the age of four to five years and can only be separated by an instrument, a trauma-inducing initial stage of surgical circumcision.

The inner layer of the prepuce has a ridged band that contains large numbers of nerve endings mediating low-threshold and fine touch sensations.[7] This ridged band area starts at the frenulum and splays out around the circumference of the inner aspect of the foreskin. When the foreskin is everted during erection, this highly sensitive structure is positioned externally for maximum pleasure during sexual activity. In the same area, there is an extensive plexus of veins and capillaries. A layer of smooth muscle bundles are oriented toward the tip of the prepuce, forming a kind of sphincter that tends to close the orifice when the penis is flaccid, preventing sand or other foreign objects from gaining access to the preputial space.

Thus, the prepuce is a uniquely sophisticated organ with highly specialized functions,[8] and is not "just a piece of skin," as advocates of mass circumcision falsely claim.

4. THE QUESTION OF MEDICAL "BENEFITS"

There is abundant literature generated in the United States on the pros and cons of neonatal circumcision. It is not surprising that *every* study alleging benefits for neonatal circumcision has been authored by an advocate for mass circumcision. The myth that circumcision is necessary to prevent penile cancer, for instance, has its origins in a 1932 article by Abraham L. Wolbarst, an early American advocate of compulsory universal circumcision.[9] Subsequently, a large number of objective scientific studies have proven this myth to be false.[10] Similarly, it has been conclusively established that male circumcision has no effect on the rate of cervical cancer in females. Other risk factors, such as early onset of sexual intercourse, multiple partners, human papilloma virus, and smoking are far more important.[11-12]

Currently, there seems to be a higher rate of urinary tract infections during the first few weeks of life among intact infants but data barely reach statistical significance. A Canadian study has concluded that 195 circumcisions would have to be performed to prevent one admission to hospital for urinary tract infection.[13] Furthermore, these researchers were only able to record a 0.12 percentage point difference in the rates of urinary tract infections between intact and circumcised infants (0.154 percent and 0.034 respectively). This difference fails to qualify as clinically significant enough to warrant the circumcision of any child.

Lately a number of studies have claimed that the risk for contracting HIV may be lower in circumcised males. Conclusive evidence, however, is still lacking, and these studies have been conducted in Africa, where confounding factors related to environment, religion, sanitary standards, and lifestyle abound.[14]

A number of professional pediatric, surgical, and obstetric societies in the United States, Canada, England, and Australia have issued statements similar to that of the American Academy of Pediatrics (AAP), namely that "these data (scientific evidence demonstrating potential medical benefits) are not sufficient to recommend routine neonatal circumcision."[15-16]

5.   COMPLICATIONS

Circumcision is alleged to be a minor operation, particularly when performed in the neonatal period and with appropriate surgical precautions. Nevertheless, the total complication rate has been found to range between two and ten percent.[17] The most common complications are bleedings and postoperative infection.[18] Other leading complications include septicemia, urinary retention, ulceration of the meatus leading to meatal stenosis, urethral fistulas, necrosis and gangrene of the glans, amputation of the entire penis, death,[19] and negative psychological sequelae.[20] Because the surgery is frequently more severe, the circumcision complication rate in third-world settings is higher.

In addition, complications from anesthesia when used may occur. Several deaths and near deaths have occurred in Sweden in recent years as a result of incompetent handling and overdosage of anesthesia and pain relievers.[21-22]

The long-term complications are less well documented. Few men are prepared to discuss their genital problems publicly. Complications subsequent to aggressive removal of the penile shaft skin have been reported to cause erectile difficulties, pain, and severe sexual problems.[23]

Another significant long-term problem relates to the fact that the circumcised penis is a religious stigma that the victim may not necessarily appreciate when he is an adult and is able to make cultural and social choices for himself. He may not wish to associate himself with the religion of his parents.

Recently, a number of circumcision malpractice cases have been brought to court in the United States where the doctor has been sued and sentenced to pay fines of up to several million dollars.[24-25]

6.   TRENDS

As mentioned above, a review of "all forms of genital mutilation and circumcision" is about to be made as part of the implementation of the Convention on the Rights of the Child. The topic is sensitive as it touches on areas of tradition and religion, which many consider to be "untouchable" areas. Yet, these issues concern the well-being of the child — a child who has no voice and no ability to refuse "treatment."

In Sweden recently, there have been a number of court cases where the Muslim father has had the circumcision executed on the son without the knowledge of or consent from the non-Muslim mother. Such cases are bound to become more common as the number of mixed marriages increase.

In Sweden, however, where, according to a leading Jewish organization in Sweden, twenty thousand Jews reside, only approximately forty percent of Jewish boys are being circumcised. The parents of the sixty percent of Jewish boys protected from circumcision presumably consider the operation dangerous, unnecessary as a religious marker, or of no importance.

In those few countries, such as the United States, Canada, Australia, and New Zealand, where policies of universal routine circumcision were implemented after World War II, there is today a definite downward trend in the rate of neonatal circumcision. In the United States, there was a peak at about ninety percent in the 1970s. It has now fallen to about fifty-seven percent. In Canada and Australia, the rate has fallen to about ten percent,[26-27] and in New Zealand, neonatal circumcision has effectively been abolished.[28] In the United Kingdom, where circumcision experienced a brief surge among the middle class in the 1930s through the early 1960s, the rate of infant circumcision has also dropped to near zero. Circumcision still persists in these countries, however, among unassimilated Muslim and Jewish immigrant groups.

7.   A NEW LAW IN SWEDEN

In 2001, the Swedish Parliament passed a law intended to regulate circumcision. Each year, approximately 3000 boys are circumcised in Sweden, but nearly all of these are born to Muslim parents. Only about forty Jewish boys are circumcised each year. During the first two months of a baby's life, a mohel (a ritual Jewish circumciser, almost always a non-physician) may perform the operation but only with a doctor (or nurse) present to give the anesthesia, which is now obligatory. The Swedish Board of Health has issued detailed instructions on how the operation is to be carried out. After two months, the operation may only be carried out by a licensed surgeon after obtaining informed consent. Inspections made recently by the Board of Health indicate that mohels are violating the terms of the new law by failing to provide the stipulated anesthesia and by circumcising boys up to four months of age.

The regulations issued by the Board of Health state that no child may be circumcised against his will — an irrelevant point because all of the children in danger of circumcision are infants or pre-school children developmentally unable to understand their predicament and unable to provide informed consent. It is furthermore mandated that, in the case of infants, the analgesic EMLA ointment, followed by infiltration local anesthesia must be used. For older children, general anesthesia or local anesthesia must be used. Mohels have only used EMLA, which is largely ineffective. Also, the surgical instruments used were sterilized but the mohels failed to indicate the expiration dates. Additionally, mohels failed to keep records of the type required for medical doctors.

In short, circumcision has been and continues to be executed "in the dark," hidden from scrutiny. Circumcision practices need to be brought out in the light, carefully scrutinized and questioned.

8. CONCLUSIONS

Female genital mutilation continues by the hundreds of thousands in many African countries and among African immigrants in the United States and Europe despite strong reactions from the United Nations and the international community, not least from women's organizations who correctly point out that this practice is incompatible with the United Nations Convention on the Rights of the Child.

Male genital mutilation, which is performed on a hundred times more victims, has attracted much less attention, although this is also incompatible with the Convention on the Rights of the Child. It is time for this unethical and medically unnecessary operation to be brought out in the light and scrutinized.

We as doctors have a clear responsibility to take a lead to start combating this primitive and brutal rite, despite its supposed "religious" origin and because of its racist function as a tool to brand a child as being different from other ethnic groups. At the very least, circumcision should be postponed until the late teenage years, when the child is legally capable of making an informed decision for himself. Similarly, circumcision could be transformed into a non-surgical symbolic rite.

It should be underscored that this "tradition" continues, in part, due to strong economic incentives. The circumcision of children is a highly lucrative venture, whether performed by American doctors, Jewish mohels, or village barbers. In the United States, circumcising doctors can net for themselves $300 just for a few minutes work.[29]

One sometimes feels ashamed to belong to the medical profession.

REFERENCES

1. Hodges FM. The ideal prepuce in ancient Greece and Rome: male genital aesthetics and their relation to lipodermos, circumcision, foreskin restoration, and the kynodesme. Bull Hist Med 2001 Fall;75(3):375-405.

2. Herodotus. History. 2.104. In: *Herodotus: The Histories*. trans. Robin Waterfield. Oxford: Oxford University Press, 1998. p. 134.

3. Glick LB. Jewish circumcision: an enigma in historical perspective. In: Understanding Circumcision: A Multi-Disciplinary Approach to a Multi-Dimensional Problem. Denniston GC, Hodges FM, Milos MF (eds). New York: Kluwer Academic/Plenum Publishers, 2001. pp. 19-54.

4. Abu-Sahlieh SA. Abu-Sahlieh SA. To mutilate in the name of Jehovah or Allah: legitimization of male and female circumcision. Med Law 1994;13(7-8):575-622.

5. Hodges FM. A short history of the institutionalization of involuntary sexual mutilation in the United States. in: Denniston GC, Milos MF (eds.), Sexual Mutilations: A Human Tragedy. New York: Plenum Press, 1997. pp. 17-40.

6. Wallerstein E. Circumcision: ritual surgery or surgical ritual? Med Law 1983;2(2):85-97.

7. Taylor JR, Lockwood AP, Taylor AJ. The prepuce: specialized mucosa of the penis and its loss to circumcision. Br J Urol 1996 Feb;77(2):291-5.

8. McGrath K. The frenular delta: a new preputial structure. In: Denniston GC, Hodges FM, Milos MF (eds). Understanding Circumcision: A Multi-Disciplinary Approach to a Multi-Dimensional Problem. New York: Kluwer Academic/Plenum Publishers, 2001. pp. 199-206.

9. Wolbarst AL. Circumcision and penile cancer. Lancet 1932 Jan 16;1(5655):150-3.

10. Circumcision policy statement. American Academy of Pediatrics. Task Force on Circumcision. Pediatrics 1999 Mar;103(3):686-93.

11. Thomas DB, Ray RM, Qin Q; The WHO Collaborative Study of Neoplasia and Steroid Contraceptives. Risk factors for progression of squamous cell cervical carcinoma in-situ to invasive cervical cancer: results of a multinational study. Cancer Causes Control 2002 Sep;13(7):683-90

12. Lehtinen M, Koskela P, Jellum E, Bloigu A, Anttila T, Hallmans G, Luukkaala T, Thoresen S, Youngman L, Dillner J, Hakama M. Herpes simplex virus and risk of cervical cancer: a longitudinal, nested case-control study in the nordic countries. Am J Epidemiol 2002 Oct 15;156(8):687-92.

13. To T, Agha M, Dick PT, Feldman W. Cohort study on circumcision of newborn boys and subsequent risk of urinary-tract infection. Lancet 1998 Dec 5;352(9143):1813-6.

14. de Vincenzi I, Mertens T. Male circumcision: a role in HIV prevention? AIDS 1994 Feb;8(2):153-60.

15. Circumcision policy statement. American Academy of Pediatrics. Task Force on Circumcision. Pediatrics 1999 Mar;103(3):686-93.

16. Fleiss PM, Hodges FM. What Your Doctor May *Not* Tell You About Circumcision. New York: Warner Books, 2002. pp. 228-30.

17. Williams N, Kapila L. Complications of circumcision. Br J Surg 1993 Oct;80(10):1231-6.

18. Kaplan GW. Complications of circumcision. Urol Clin North Am 1983 Aug;10(3):543-9.

19. Fleiss PM, Hodges FM. What Your Doctor May *Not* Tell You About Circumcision. New York: Warner Books, 2002. pp. 76-9.

20. Boyle GJ, Bensley GA. Adverse sexual and psychological effects of male infant circumcision. Psychol Rep 2001 Jun;88(3 Pt 2):1105-6.

21. Hofvander Y, Olsen L. [Circumcision of boys — a child's right versus parents' right]. Lakartidningen 2000 May 24;97(21):2598-604.

22. Hofvander Y. New law on male circumcision in Sweden. Lancet 2002 Feb 16;359(9306):630.

23. Peterson SE. Assaulted and mutilated. A personal account of circumcision trauma. In: Denniston GC, Hodges FM, Milos MF (eds). Understanding Circumcision: A Multi-Disciplinary Approach to a Multi-Dimensional Problem. New York: Kluwer Academic/Plenum Publishers, 2001. pp. 271-89.

24. Huff D. Youth gets $1.5 million for bungled operations. Arizona Daily Star. (August 1990).

25. Associated Press. $1.4M awarded for botched circumcision. Santa Cruz Sentinel (9 June 2001): p. A5. cited in: Fleiss PM, Hodges FM. What Your Doctor May *Not* Tell You About Circumcision. New York: Warner Books, 2002. p. 139.

26. Association for Genital Integrity. Circumcision rates in Canada. URL: http://www.courtchallenge.com/refs/rate1m.html

27. Williams G. NOCIRC of Australia. In: Denniston GC, Milos MF (eds). Sexual Mutilations: A Human Tragedy. New York: Plenum Press, 1997. pp. 189-95.

28. McGrath K, Young H. A review of circumcision in New Zealand: 'I never liked doing them and I was pleased to give them up'. In: Denniston GC, Hodges FM, Milos MF (eds). Understanding Circumcision: A Multi-Disciplinary Approach to a Multi-Dimensional Problem. New York: Kluwer Academic/Plenum Publishers, 2001. pp. 129-46.

29. Fletcher CR. Circumcision in America in 1998: attitudes, beliefs, and charges of American physicians. In: Denniston GC, Hodges FM, Milos MF (eds.). Males and Female Circumcision: Medical, Legal, and Ethical Considerations in Pediatrics Practice. New York: Kluwer Academic/Plenum Publishers, 1999. pp. 259-71.

Chapter 10

ANTHROPOLOGY AND FEMALE GENITAL CUTTING (FGC)
What Took Us So Long to Come Around?

Marianne M. Sarkis, MA
University of South Florida, Department of Child and Family Studies, Louis de la Parte Mental Health Institute. Director, Female Genital Mutilation Awareness and Education Project of NOCIRC

Abstract: Because of their relativistic stance, anthropologists have been harshly criticized by activists both inside and outside the discipline for failing to take a stance on the issue of female genital cutting (FGC). In the last five years, the approach taken by some anthropologists has been more critical and questioning, emphasizing the need to return to empirical research and data gathering because there are many unknowns left in the body of literature and any stance taken has to be a result of this research. In this paper, I will explore some of these recent developments and studies, all the while trying to reconcile cultural relativism and the holistic approach of anthropology with that of advocacy and activism.

Key words: Female genital mutilation, circumcision, anthropology

1. INTRODUCTION

When I was fourteen, growing up in Lebanon, I came across a book entitled *Women: Why do you Weep?* by Asma El Dareer.[1] The book discussed the practice of female genital cutting (FGC). At the time, the practice was not discussed in polite company.[2] I was so moved by what I read, that I decided to dedicate my life to working for the eradication of the practice. When it was time for me to start college in the United States, I needed to find an academic major that would allow me to focus on the study of this practice, while maintaining my activism and my sense and drive to

Flesh and Blood, Edited by Denniston et al.
Kluwer Academic/Plenum Publishers, New York 2004

119

work on its eradication. The closest I was able to get was the field of anthropology. My reasoning was that, since anthropology was the study of other cultures and their practices, my focus on female cutting and initiation rites would not be considered out of the ordinary. My belief, at the time, was that I could find support for my work in anthropology. Little did I know how intellectually and politically challenging that decision would be. In the next few years, as an undergraduate and graduate student, almost every paper I presented on the issue was returned with either a "too controversial" or "too focused" comment. I was encouraged to focus on something else, such as poverty, women's reproductive health, or the status of women in Africa and the Middle East. Until very recently, I did not understand why that was the case. Why, in a cutting-edge field like anthropology, would professors and mentors actively try to dissuade me from focusing on this important issue. I knew the answer would have to be in the much-strained relationship between anthropology and human rights, and between human rights and activism.

2.   ANTHROPOLOGY AND CULTURAL RELATIVISM

One of the core tenets of anthropology is the idea of "cultural relativism." It is argued that all cultures should be considered equal, and that no one culture is superior to any other. As anthropologists, our study of other cultures should be free of bias and judgment in order to allow objective observations and recording.

As a result, until very recently, organized anthropological associations have actively stayed out of discussions that endorse human rights resolutions such as the Universal Declaration of Human Rights, which was passed in 1947 by the United Nations, because they believed that "no such declaration would be applicable to all human beings."[3] Consequently, the anthropological point of view was absent from subsequent discussions and resolutions such as the United Nations "Convention on the Elimination of All Forms of Discrimination Against Women," which was approved in 1979.

This is not to say that anthropologists have been completely absent from testifying and speaking out about atrocities, such as the holocaust and apartheid. However, when it comes to violence against individual rights, such as those involving women and children, they have not taken a stance.

In this paper, I will outline some early approaches anthropologists used to look at FGC. Next, I will focus on the West's academic and media reactions in the wake of exposure to the practice. Then, I will briefly look at the way the United Nations has attempted to support various eradication efforts.

The final section of my paper will focus on anthropology's relativistic stance and some of the criticisms it has faced as a result, and the way I believe applied anthropologists have recently stepped up to the challenge of becoming more involved in both research and activism, concluding with some current research and encouraging results that show positive changes and a decrease in numbers of women affected by FGC.

3.   FEMALE GENITAL CUTTING AND THE WEST

The earliest mentions of FGC in the general literature appeared in regional medical journals,[4-8] explorers correspondences,[9] local and regional studies,[10-14] and topical research mostly focusing on initiation rites.[15-20] These early references portrayed FGC as an initiation rite or an exotic practice.[21] Descriptions were mostly objective and clinical without much social and cultural contextualization.[22]

In 1935, Jomo Kenyatta, a student of Bronislaw Malinowski and later the president of Kenya, argued strongly in favor of female circumcision in the Kikuyu tribes. He viewed British efforts to outlaw the practice as another form of Imperialism.[23] He believed that FGC had positive social value and was a symbol of national identity.[24] Kenyatta asserts:

> The real anthropological study, therefore, is to show that clitoridectomy, like Jewish circumcision, is a mere bodily mutilation which, however, is regarded as the conditio sine qua non of the whole teaching of tribal law, religion, and morality.

> The initiation of both sexes is the most important custom among the Gikuyu . It is looked upon as a deciding factor in giving a boy or girl the status of manhood or womanhood in the Gikuyu community. This custom is adhered to by the vast majority of African peoples and is found in almost every part of the continent. It is therefore necessary to examine the facts attached to this widespread custom in order to have some idea why the African peoples cling to this custom which, in the eyes of a good many Europeans, is nothing but a "horrible" and "painful" practice, suitable only to barbarians.[25]

With the rise of feminist theory in the 1970s, female circumcision began receiving international attention from academics and activists. The tone at the time was combative, and placed the practice in a context of the global oppression of women and the domineering patriarchy. This is illustrated by Mary Daly's chapter on "African Genital Mutilations: The Unspeakable Atrocities" in her book, *Gyn-Ecology*:

There are some manifestations of the Sado-Ritual Syndrome that are unspeakable – incapable of being expressed in words because they are inexpressibly horrible. Such are the ritual of genital mutilations – excision and infibulation – still inflicted upon women throughout Africa today, and practiced in many parts of the world in the past.[26]

During this time, many articles describing the horrors of FGC practices appeared in magazines and newspapers with titles such as "International Crime,"[27] "Unspeakable Atrocities,"[28] "Victims of Tradition,"[29] and "Prisoners of Ritual."[30] This literary uproar alienated Third World feminists from their Western colleagues, culminating in the threat of a walkout by a group of African activists during the International Women's Conference in Copenhagen in 1980.[31] Third World activists saw the Western international outcry against FGC practices as another form of cultural imperialism.[32-33]

In 1980, *Ms. Magazine* published an article by Nawal el Saadawi, a leading Egyptian feminist physician, along with an accompanying article by Gloria Steinem and Robin Morgan,[34] that exposed FGC to the Western media[35] and brought international attention to the practice. Like Daly,[36] the practice was placed in a patriarchal framework devoid of any cultural significance.

Also, during this time, African and Arab women began to raise their own voices about their experiences.[37-41] As Third World activists tried to devise ways to eradicate FGC and gain financial and in-kind support from international agencies, the debate with First World feminists increased and became more heated. The common thread in much of the Western-biased literature was the characterization of African and Arab women as victims of "patriarchy, ignorance, or both."[42] These views are still prevalent in 1990s literature on this topic. Some examples include Alice Walker and Pratibha Parmar's book, *Warrior Marks*,[43] the 1993 documentary of the same title, and a special edition on FGC published by the National Organization for Women (NOW).[44]

Though *Warrior Marks* resulted in increased awareness of FGC, it tried to appeal to the West with a sensationalized picture of African women "mutilated and sexually blinded" by unquestioned traditions and male domination.[45] Again, much like the pre-1980s approach, the custom was presented in a context devoid of cultural and symbolic significance. Walley notes that:

> [T]his frustrating sense of déjà vu may be dismissed as Walker's and NOW's refusal to engage the productive aspects of earlier debates. However, more pertinent to understanding why these accounts have generated such a barrage of media attention is the way that Walker's and NOW's presentation of female genital operations have fed into powerful and value-laden understandings of differences between Africans and Euro-Americans – understandings that are

being reemphasized with increased immigration from the Third World to the First…Reading through much of the Western-based literature opposing female genital operations, the degree to which many of the arguments work to reproduce such beliefs is striking.[46]

As a result of some of the subsequent conferences on FGC, numerous African women's organizations raised the issue of FGC to a high priority. Work to establish ways of eradicating the practice locally and across Africa began. In 1984, the Inter-African Committee Against Traditional Practices Affecting the Health of Women and Children NGO (IAC) was formed, with regional and national affiliates in twenty-three African countries.[47] In addition, the World Health Organization "gave its name and credibility to NGOs and campaigners working directly in the field."[48] In Kenya, the women's organization, Maendeleo ya Wanawake (The Development of Women), also was formed in the 1980s to develop community-based programs to eliminate FGC. In Uganda, the Reproductive, Educative and Community Health Programme has a similar agenda, while offering alternative initiation rites to women and midwives.[49] In Ghana, the Association of Church Development Projects (ACDEP) was formed, with aims[goals that included???], including "programmes on research, training and rehabilitation, public awareness, legislation and coordination of efforts."[50]

The United Nations and many of its affiliates (e.g., UNICEF and WHO) attempted to draw up concise resolutions and charters that would clearly state their position on the issue of FGC. Anastasios Zavales, Secretary-General of Ecumenics International, notes that FGC violates over eighteen United Nations charters and resolutions.[51] So far, these do not seem to be very effective in eradicating FGC because they fail to consider a holistic view of the practice. For example, the *Declaration of the Rights of the Child* asserts that states parties shall take all appropriate measures to ensure that the child is protected against all forms of discrimination or punishment on the basis of the status, activities, expressed opinions, or beliefs of the child's parents, legal guardians, or family members."[52]

This ambiguity and the idealistic attitude of this resolution make it difficult to enforce. In other words, what determines "discrimination or punishment?" Who determines them and why? Furthermore, similar resolutions fail to take into consideration the fact that many people in remote villages and deserts of Africa and the Middle East are simply unaware of what constitutes a "human right."[53] The issues of human "right" and protection of the child are very difficult to determine. These questions would have benefited from the anthropological perspective, which seeks to address such issues as they apply to different cultures.

4.   ANTHROPOLOGICAL CONTRIBUTIONS TO THE STUDY OF FGC

Regarding cultural relativism, Erve Chambers explains that a relativistic perspective is important to anthropologists because it encourages them to make sense of a social or cultural situation from a position of value impartiality. This *does* (why italics?] not mean that the anthropologist must necessarily withhold judgment about the conduct of human affairs, but only that his or her judgment is best informed by an impartial view of the cultural antecedents to specific human behavior and values."[54]

However, because of their relativistic stance, anthropologists have taken a long time to address issues of eradication and advocacy regarding FGC, and, as a result, have been harshly criticized by activists both within and without the discipline. For example, in 1982, Fran Hosken criticized anthropologists for engaging in what she called a "cover-up" on the issue of FGC and its harmful effects. She states:

> Anthropologists and sociologists have failed to report the health damage involved in the practices they describe in their literature. One can read today descriptions of the colorful initiation rites, including excision, without one word about the tortures and mutilations, and the permanent health damage that these brutal procedures involved which young children are forced to undergo, either by social pressure or by physical force. The victims of the practices described here are for the most part illiterate and too young to speak for themselves, unaware of the rest of the world and of their own bodies' biological functions.[55]

In a conversation with Ms. Hosken, I had an opportunity to explain what 'applied anthropology' means, and how it can be useful in helping international efforts to eradicate FGC on the national and international level. Ms. Hosken was unaware of such a field and refused to listen to my explanation. I think her attitude reflects a general belief that anthropology is paralyzed by a "cultural relativism" stance,[56] and another feminist noted that "anthropologists are unlikely to wield any direct influence in the current debate, whether or not they abandon their relativist stance."[57]

In its most basic definition, applied anthropology is "the activity of professional anthropologists in programs that, as primary goals, have changes in human behavior believed to ameliorate contemporary social, economic, and technological problems."[58] In other words, applied anthropologists work with local communities to become change agents.

As the FGC debate commenced, and anthropologists attempted to make sense out of this difficult issue, Simon Messing, one of the forefathers of applied anthropology, advised that applied anthropologists cannot evade the issue of such a serious and widespread problem as genital mutilation of females if they are concerned with public health. The problem is growing with the increase in population in the so-called less developed countries. It is also entering a further new dimension when these medically useless and traumatic operations are increasingly adopted by government-supervised hospitals, which thereby imply their approval. If applied anthropologists are to have a chance to participate in rational and responsible planning in the development of public health, they should not leave the burden of this task entirely on the shoulders of radical feminists – and the latter in turn should welcome our cooperation.[59]

Until quite recently, applied anthropology literature concerning FGC was scarce. After surveying *Human Organization, Anthropology Newsletter,* and *Practicing Anthropology*, I have found less than five anthropologists (and no applied anthropologists) published in them.

Anthropologists struggled to understand the practice of FGC by placing it in its proper socio-cultural context. Elizabeth Hicks[60] wrote about the economic significance of infibulation in Africa while Janice Boddy[61] wrote about the symbolic significance of female circumcision in the Sudan. In 1982, Ellen Gruenbaum[62] also tried to evaluate and observe the movement against FGC in the Sudan. She attempted to point out the significance and the context of this practice not only as an initiation rite, but also as an ethnic, religious, familial, and gender-based marker.[63]

In 1982, Fran Hosken published the first of her reports on FGC in Africa and the Middle East. *The Hosken Report*[64] went unchallenged until the early 1990s. An architect by training and no proper anthropological instruction, Hosken traveled extensively throughout Africa and the Middle East and "reported" on the incidences of FGC. Her findings were the only reports readily available at the time. Her data went unrefuted until ten years ago when anthropologists, activists, and medical professionals started reporting their own findings.

It wasn't until 1999 that an anthropologist directly questioned Hosken's reports, taking issue with her data concerning the extent of the practice and her records on the physical and psychological effects of FGC.[65] Obermeyer dismisses the *Hosken Report* because of the "poor quality of the evidence [it uses], and the methodological shortcomings of [its] estimations."[66] In addition, Obermeyer finally states what many anthropologists had been struggling to say until that point:

> [T]hat the evidence has been until now long on advocacy and short on empirically based research reflects the prominence of the concerns of activists in guiding the research agenda, and the disproportional allocation of resources toward 'intervention studies' aimed at abolishing the practice, rather than toward scientific inquiry.[67]

What Obermeyer acknowledged in the previous statement was that anthropologists have neglected to question some of the data published on this issue; and that they have derived their assessments and evaluations from these data at the expense of gaining empirical knowledge first-hand. Obermeyer's liberating statement was a call to action on behalf of anthropologists, especially applied anthropologists. Two years later, two books were finally published in applied anthropology regarding FGC and the role of anthropology.

Ellen Gruenbaum's book, *The Female Circumcision Controversy: An Anthropological Perspective,*[68] was the culmination of twenty-five years of work in the Sudan and other parts of Africa. In her introduction, she outlines the development of her stance and her struggle to understand this practice moving from a purely theoretical perspective of cultural relativism to an applied perspective.

Bettina Shell-Duncan and Ylva Hernlund's book, *Female 'Circumcision' in Africa: Culture, Controversy and Change,*[69] was published by Lynne Reinner Publications as part of the *Directions in Applied Anthropology* series. This book originated from a panel that I organized at the 1997 Annual Meeting of the Society for Applied Anthropology in Seattle, Washington. The goal of this book is to observe the practice of FGC in a cultural context. The result is almost an answer to Gruenbaum's position that "the peoples affected are arguing this out for themselves."[70] *Female 'Circumcision' in Africa* is primarily a compilation of articles written by activists, physicians, feminists, and Western anthropologists practicing in areas affected by FGC within Africa and the Middle East.

FGC provides an interesting challenge to anthropology, and especially to applied anthropology. Anthropologists must adhere to a cultural relativism stance, but applied anthropologists also have a responsibility to offer a helping hand when the opportunity presents itself.

In the last five years, the approach taken by some anthropologists has been more critical and questioning, emphasizing the need to return to empirical research and data gathering as there are many unknowns left in the body of literature.[71] Ellen Gruenbaum[72] seems quite enthusiastic and hopeful of the current trends developing in anthropology regarding the practice of FGC and its surrounding issues. While still advocating the "hands-off approach,"[73] she now admits that anthropologists have much to offer regarding research as well as a critical assessment of traditional practices affecting the health of women and children. She notes:

> [R]ecent analytical work and public education writing by anthropologists (and our kindred social scientists) has developed in a very gratifying direction, generally offering the contextualized analyses while accepting and contributing to ideas for change...[recent body of literature] offer examples of contextualized

analysis that neither condemns those who practice female circumcision nor endorses the continuation. This new body of literature could perhaps be characterized as being calm and optimistic about the prospects for change, while urging critics and reformers to make serious attempts to understand the contexts."[74]

5.   ARE FGC CHANGES ON THE HORIZON?

While researching the relationship of anthropology and FGC regarding female genital operations, the majority of the articles written on the topic in the last twenty years in the anthropological literature focused on two main issues:

How can anthropology come to a culturally sensitive understanding with this issue that leaves room for cultural negotiation for change?

Why haven't anthropologists been more involved in the struggle to abandon this practice?

Unlike literature in the general media, the articles in the anthropological journals and books were descriptive of the practices and dealt mostly with an ongoing struggle to place the issue of FGC in a larger context such as maternal health, gender identity, human rights, and other theoretical paradigms.

The surprising issue that came out of this review is the lack of material that dealt with any types of advocacy or action. Except for some recent studies,[75-77] anthropologists reported stories about witnessing these practices, but very few of them reported getting actively involved in trying to help in its eradication. Gruenbaum notes that, "although anthropologists may passionately oppose female circumcision, I believe the most useful role is to provide cultural perspectives on it, offer a sophisticated analysis of why these practices continue, and describe the forces for change in various cultural contexts."[78]

This force for change, while slow in progress and effect, needs to take into consideration not only the immediate effects of FGC in a culture, but also the context in which it exists. For example, a successful program in the Gambia, "the ritual without cutting,"[79] demonstrates this point. This is a program that understands the importance of female cutting as an initiatory rite and attempts to replace it with other rituals that do not involve cutting and bleeding. This would still allow the transmission of knowledge that usually takes place during the ritual without the harmful effects that accompany FGC.

Another successful program in Mali not only takes into consideration the girls who are being cut but also the midwives, whose sole financial livelihood is the money that comes from circumcising. Various NGOs have taken on successful programs of "handing over the knife" programs.[80] An example of this program took place in Mali and did just that. Claudie Gosselin describes her work with a Malian organization whose purpose was to rehabilitate traditional excisers in other income-generating activities, after they hand over their knives in a public ceremony. Gosselin notes that "Aid donors, foreign feminists, and human rights activists working to end excision often do not have the benefit of this knowledge. Such an understanding, however, allows one to apprehend the local meanings associated with the practice of excision and the social status of those who perform it."[81]

These programs, while NGO driven, are developed from within the cultures affected, but also, in some cases, with the help of foreign aid donors, feminists, and activists. The two operate hand-in-hand. Everything we do as outsiders must take place in support and in a "hands-off" manner that Gruenbaum[82] advocates.

Especially of note here is that uniform solutions to this issue are not reasonable because they don't allow for the multiplicity of experiences, types, and reasons of FGC, and the reasons why cultures still hold on to them. This echoes Mandara's view that:

Successful change requires not only understanding but also appreciation of the reasons for sustaining the practice. Only by offering alternative ways of achieving the same objective can we hope to completely and permanently eradicate female genital cutting.[83]

REFERENCES

1. El Dareer A. Woman, why do you weep?: circumcision and its consequences. London: Zed Press, 1982.
2. Gruenbaum E. The female circumcision controversy: An Anthropological Perspective. Philadelphia: University of Pennsylvania Press, 2001. [here, p. 21.]
3. Flueher-Lobaan C. Cultural relativism and universal rights. The Chronicle of Higher Education (9 June 1985): p. 9.
4. Dewhurst CJ. Infibulation complicating pregnancy. British Medical Journal 1964;2:1442.
5. Huddleston CE. Female circumcision in the Sudan. Lancet 1949;1:626.
6. Laycock HT. Surgical aspects of female circumcision in Somaliland. East African Medical Journal 1950;27:445-50.
7. Meuwissen JHJM. Human infertility in west Africa. Tropical and Geographic Medicine 1966;18:147-52.
8. Sequira JH. Female circumcision and infibulation. Lancet 1931;2:1054-1056.
9. Orde-Browne G. Circumcision ceremonies among the Amwimbe. Man 1913;79:137-40.
10. Butt-Thompson FW. West African secret societies. London: H.F. and G. Witherby; 1929.
11. Dieterlen G. Essai sur la religion Bambara. Paris: Presses Universitaires de France; 1951.
12. Griaule M. Conversations with Ogotenmeli: An introduction to Dogon religious ideas. London: Oxford University Press, 1965.

13. Leakey LSB. The Kikuyu problem of the initiation of girls. Journal of the Royal Anthropological Institute of Great Britain and Ireland 1931;61:277-85.

14. Meek CK. The Northern tribes of Nigeria. Oxford: Oxford University Press; 1925.

15. Bethelheim B. Symbolic wounds: Puberty rites and the envious male. New York: Collier Books; 1962.

16. Bonaparte M. Female sexuality. New York: International Universities Press; 1953.

17. Bryk F. Circumcision in man and woman: Its history, psychology and ethnology. New York: American Ethnological Press; 1934.

18. Orde-Brown GJ. Circumcision ceremonies among the Amwimbe. Man 1913;79:137-40.

19. Van Gennep AV. The rites of passage. Chicago: University of Chicago Press;1960.

20. Widstrand CG. Female infibulation. Occasional Papers of Studia Ethnographica Upsaliensia 1964;20:95-124.

21. Bryk F. Circumcision in man and woman: Its history, psychology and ethnology. New York: American Ethnological Press;1934.

22. Gruenbaum E. The female circumcision controversy: An anthropological perspective. Philadelphia: University of Pennsylvania Press; 2001.

23. Gruenbaum E. The female circumcision controversy: An anthropological perspective. Philadelphia: University of Pennsylvania Press, 2001. [here, p. 25.]

24. Gruenbaum E. The female circumcision controversy: An anthropological perspective. Philadelphia: University of Pennsylvania Press, 2001. [here, p. 207.]

25. Kenyatta J. Facing Mt. Kenya: The tribal life of the Kikuyu. New York: Vintage Books, 1965. [here, p. 125.]

26. Daly M. Gyn-ecology: The metaethics of radical feminism. Boston: Beacon Press, 1978. [here, p. 155.]

27. Morgan R, Steinem G. The international crime of genital mutilation. Ms. 1980;8(9):65-7.

28. Daly M. Gyn-ecology: The metaethics of radical feminism. Boston: Beacon Press, 1978.

29. Mays S, Stockley A. Victims of tradition. Nursing Mirror 1983;156:19-21.

30. Lightfoot-Klein H. Prisoners of ritual: An odyssey into female genital circumcision in Africa. New York: Harrington Park Press;1989.

31. Walley CJ. Searching for 'voices': feminism, anthropology, and the global debate over female genital operations. Cultural Anthropology 1997;12:405-38. [here, p. 419.]

32. Thomburn KM. To combat FGM, African women should lead and we should follow. Physicians for Human Rights Record [serial online]. 1996 May [cited 2002 April 13]; ix(1):[21 screens] Available from: URL: http://www.phrusa.org/about/PHRRmay96.html

33. Morsy S. Safeguarding women's bodies: the white man's burden medicalized. Medical Anthropology Quarterly 1991;5:19-23.

34. Morgan R., Steinem G. The international crime of genital mutilation. Ms. 1980;8(9):65-7.

35. El Saadawi N. The question no one would answer. Ms. 1980;8(9):64.

36. Daly M. Gyn-ecology: The metaethics of radical feminism. Boston: Beacon Press, 1978.

37. El Saadawi N. The hidden face of eve: women in the Arab world. London: Zed Press; 1980.

38. Abdalla RHD. Sisters in affliction: circumcision and infibulation of women in Africa. London: Zed Press, 1982.

39. El Dareer A. Woman, why do you weep? Circumcision and its consequences. London: Zed Press, 1982.

40. Toubia N. The social and political implications of female circumcision: The case of Sudan. In: Fernea EW, editor. Women and the family in the Middle East: New voices of Change. Austin: University of Texas Press, 1985. pp. 148-59

41. Thiam A. Black sisters, speak out: Feminism and oppression in black Africa. London: Pluto, 1986.

42. Walley CJ. Searching for 'voices': feminism, anthropology, and the global debate over female genital operations. Cultural Anthropology 1997;12:405-38. [here, p. 419.]
43. Walker A, Parmar P. Warrior marks: female genital mutilation and the sexual blinding of women. New York: Harcourt Brace, 1993.
44. National Organization for Women (NOW). Newsletter special supplement on female genital mutilation. 1996.
45. Gruenbaum E. The female circumcision controversy: An anthropological perspective. Philadelphia: University of Pennsylvania Press, 2001. [here, p. 23.]
46. Walley CJ. Searching for 'voices': feminism, anthropology, and the global debate over female genital operations. Cultural Anthropology 1997;12:405-38. [here, p. 419.]
47. Toubia N. Female genital mutilation: a call for global action. New York: Rainbow/Women Ink, 1995.
48. Dorkenoo E. Combating female genital mutilation: an agenda for the next decade. World Health Statistics Quarterly 1996;49:142-7.
49. Sadik N. Statement. Conference of African women ministers and parliamentaries; 1996 Oct 25-28 [cited 2002 April 13]; Dar Es Salaam, Khartoum. Available from: URL: gopher://gopher.undp.org/00/ungophers/popin/unfpa/speeches/1996/tanzania.txt
50. Amnesty International. Working together for change to stop female genital mutilation. Collaborative programme of Amnesty International-Ghana & the Association of Church Development Projects (ACDEP) in Northern Ghana Treasury Conference Centre, Bolgatanga, Upper-East Region, Ghana. 1996.
51. Zavales A. The international human rights challenge of genital mutilation & the United Nations. New York:Ecumenics International Press, 1994. [here, p. 6.]
52. Zavales A. The international human rights challenge of genital mutilation & the United Nations. New York:Ecumenics International Press, 1994. [here, p. 32.]
53. Hosken F. Personal communication. 1995.
54. Chambers E. Applied anthropology. Englewood Cliffs, NJ: Prentice Hall, 1985. [here, p. 3.]
55. Hosken F. The Hosken report: Genital and sexual mutilation of females, 3d ed. Lexington, Mass.: Women's International Network News, 1982. [here, p. 6.]
56. Gordon D. Female circumcision and genital operations in Egypt and the Sudan: A Dilemma for medical anthropology. Med Anthropol Q 1991;1:3-14. [here, p. 13.]
57. Lyons H. Anthropologists, moralities, and relativities: The problem of genital mutilations. Canadian Review of Sociology and Anthropology. 1981;18:499-518. [here, p. 514.]
58. Anthromorphemics: Anthropology Glossary. Available from: URL: http://www.anth.ucsb.edu/glossary
59. Messing S. The problem of operations based on custom in applied anthropology: The challenge of the Hosken report on genital and sexual mutilations of females. Human Organization 1980;39:295-7. [here, p. 297.]
60. Hicks EK. Infibulation: Female mutilation in Islamic Northeastern Africa. New Brunswick: Transaction Publishers, 1982.
61. Boddy J. Womb as oasis: The symbolic content of pharaonic circumcision in rural Northern Sudan. American Ethnologist 1982;9:682-98.
62. Gruenbaum E. The movement against clitoridectomy and infibulation in Sudan: Public health policy and the women's Movement. Medical Anthropology Newsletter 1982;13(2):4-12.
63. Gruenbaum E. The female circumcision controversy: An anthropological perspective. Philadelphia: University of Pennsylvania Press, 2001.
64. Hosken F. The Hosken report: genital and sexual mutilation of females, 3d ed. Lexington, Mass: Women's International Network News, 1982.

65. Obermeyer CM. Female genital surgeries: The known, the unknown, and the unknowable,. Med Anthropol Q 1999;13(1):79-106.
66. Obermeyer CM. Female genital surgeries: The known, the unknown, and the unknowable,. Med Anthropol Q 1999;13(1):79-106. [here, p. 84.]
67. Obermeyer CM. Female genital surgeries: The known, the unknown, and the unknowable,. Med Anthropol Q 1999;13(1):79-106. [here, p. 85.]
68. Gruenbaum E. The female circumcision controversy: An anthropological perspective. Philadelphia: University of Pennsylvania Press; 2001.
69. Shell-Duncan B, Hernlund Y, editors. Female circumcision in Africa: Culture, controversy, and change. Boulder, CO: Lynne Rienner Publishers, 2001.
70. Gruenbaum E. The female circumcision controversy: An anthropological perspective. Philadelphia: University of Pennsylvania Press, 2001. [here, p. 23.]
71. Walley CJ. Searching for 'voices': Feminism, anthropology, and the global debate over female genital operations. Cultural Anthropology 1997;12:405-38.
72. Gruenbaum E. The female circumcision controversy: An anthropological perspective. Philadelphia: University of Pennsylvania Press, 2001.
73. Gruenbaum E. The cultural debate over female circumcision: The Sudanese Are Arguing This One Out for Themselves. Med Anthropol Q 1996;10:455-75.
74. Gruenbaum E. The female circumcision controversy: An anthropological perspective. Philadelphia: University of Pennsylvania Press, 2001. [here, p. 23.]
75. Gruenbaum E. The cultural debate over female circumcision: the Sudanese are arguing this one out for themselves. Med Anthropol Q 1996;10:455-75.
76. Gruenbaum E. The female circumcision controversy: An anthropological perspective. Philadelphia: University of Pennsylvania Press, 2001.
77. Shell-Duncan B, Hernlund Y, editors. Female circumcision in Africa: Culture, controversy, and change. Boulder, CO: Lynne Rienner Publishers, 2001.
78. Gruenbaum E. The cultural debate over female circumcision: the Sudanese are arguing this one out for themselves. Med Anthropol Q 1996; 10:455-75. [here, p. 456.]
79. Hernlund Y. Cutting without ritual and ritual without cutting: female "circumcision" and the re-ritualization of initiation in the Gambia? In: Shell-Duncan B, Herlund Y, editors. Female circumcision in Africa: Culture, controversy, and change. Boulder (CO): Lynne Rienner Publishers, 2000. pp. 235-52.
80. Gosselin C. Handing over the knife: Numu women and the campaign against excision in Mali. In: Shell-Duncan B, Hernlund Y, editors. Female circumcision in Africa: Culture, controversy, and change. Boulder (CO): Lynne Rienner Publishers, 2000. pp. 167-92.
81. Gosselin C. Handing over the knife: Numu women and the campaign against excision in Mali. In: Shell-Duncan B, Hernlund Y, editors. Female circumcision in Africa: Culture, controversy, and change. Boulder (CO): Lynne Rienner Publishers, 2000. pp. 167-92. [here, p. 192.]
82. Gruenbaum E. The cultural debate over female circumcision: the Sudanese are arguing this one out for themselves. Med Anthropol Q 1996;10:455-75.
83. Mandara MU. Female genital cutting in Nigeria: Views of Nigerian doctors on the medicalization debate. In: Shell-Duncan B, Hernlund Y, editors. Female circumcision in Africa: Culture, controversy, and change. Boulder (CO): Lynne Rienner Publishers, 2000. pp. 95-108.

Chapter 11

CHANGES IN INFIBULATION PRACTICE IN EAST AFRICA

Comments on a Ritual Alternative to Infibulation in Merka, Somalia

Pia Grassivaro Gallo, Ph.D., Marica Livio, Ph.D., Franco Viviani, Ph.D.
Faculty of Psychology, University of Padua, Italy

Abstract: According to the available information from Somalia and Sudan, female infibulation in East Africa is moving more toward *sunna* rather than its complete eradication. In Merka, Somalia, *sunna* has evolved into a unique practice called *sunna gudnin*. A videotape, shot on location in Somalia, has been used as an educational and therapeutic tool to promote the idea of non-circumcision. From 1999 to 2001, the videotape was presented at international congresses and meetings on female genital mutilation (London, Ghent, Sydney), where Somalis working on international projects on immigration were in attendance. In Italy, the videotape was shown to Somali social workers in Rome and Padua, to Sudanese students visiting the University of Padua, and to students at the University of Padua in the Faculties of Psychology and Agricultural Science. From the discussions that ensue following each presentation of the video, we conclude that the *sunna gudnin* ritual, as well as other alternatives to female genital mutilation, are acceptable to the populations that devised them, but cannot be exported to other populations.

Key words: Circumcision, female genital mutilation, infibulation, *sunna gudnin*, Somalia,

1.   INFIBULATION IN EAST AFRICA TODAY

Alternative ceremonies to female genital mutilation (FGM) have already been described in a previous paper.[1] We would now like to consider the evolution of infibulation in East Africa, looking specifically at two countries, Sudan and Somalia, where the custom persists.

In the Sudan, Dr. Amna A.R. Hassan,[2-3] who is the Executive Secretary of the Sudan National Committee on Harmful Traditional Practices (SNCTP) in the Khartoum North and East Nile Provinces, carried out an important in-depth study over four years (1996 to 2000). This study was sponsored by SNCTP and "Save the Children," Sweden. A statistical approach was used, together with various tools (questionnaires, interviews, observation, the Participatory Rapid Appraisal, focus group discussions, etc.). The random sample included teenagers of both sexes (1,000 subjects), aged eighteen, plus 230 parents of female pupils, and 160 midwives (between twenty-eight and seventy-five years of age). The most important findings of the study were that infibulation practices are more widespread than the so-called *sunna* type circumcision amongst Muslims (ninety-seven and eighty-eight percent in rural areas and in the urban areas respectively).

Regarding the attitude to change the ritual, seventy-three percent of the sample agreed to continue with *sunna* and twenty-seven percent supported infibulation.

There was a marked recent transformation of the tradition from infibulation to *sunna*; prevalence of the female pupils: fifty-seven percent and forty-three percent in favor of infibulation and *sunna*, respectively; in the case of their mothers: eighty-five percent and fifteen percent. The data were also confirmed by a group of Sudanese students interviewed in Padua (summer 2001). A clear tendency towards attenuation in the practice, however, appears to be limited to the capital city, since it was not confirmed for the rural regions. Moreover, the capital is also the home of the Ahfad University for Women, based in Ondurman, a private institution dedicated to providing girls with a basic education. The university involves its female students in practical activities, thereby giving them the opportunity to measure themselves against social realities. The university is a powerful force for change in the status of females. After the Khartoum Conference (1979), the University instituted the Babiker Bedri Scientific Association for Women's Studies, which is working towards the eradication of the infibulation.[4] This Association works with the support of the Ministry of Health, organizing specific seminars for the different ethnic groups, but continues to recommend *sunna* for those families who are unwilling to break away from tradition completely.[5]

For areas outlying the capital city, Ellen Gruenbaum carried out a study investigating links between health educators, innovators, and rural populations.[6] She issued the first significant report on the Abdal Galil region, a rural center with a fairly high economic level due to the fact that members of many families work in the town. Here, the rural medical assistant in charge of the Health Center began introducing health education to all sectors because he strongly believed in prevention and in promoting public health measures. Regarding female circumcision, he was convinced of its harmfulness for four reasons: it is bad, not Islamic, sinful, and it causes difficult births. He promoted and organized single-sex meetings in schools, without great success, it must be said. His highest priority was to change men's opinions. His activities, however, were significant because he prepared the public to accept an evolution in the practice of infibulation. Following this man's efforts, an increasing number of traditional medical assistants began to take a stand against infibulation. In fact, from 1970 to the early 1990s, the most severe form of circumcision was progressively abandoned in favor of *sunna*. New forms of mildly invasive circumcision were developed, such as one proposed by a well-respected traditional nurse. Working in the main town of Wad Medani province, she carried out circumcisions, assisted childbirth, and performed minor surgery. The form of mutilation she practiced left the clitoris intact but sewn beneath a small flap of tissue. In this way, though not explicitly condemning infibulation, this nurse disseminated and supported milder forms of excision. Her intervention, a particular form of *sunna*, removed only a small part of the prepuce, leaving erectile tissue intact, safeguarding sexual sensitivity, and reducing the possibility of the patient contracting the most common post-operative communicable diseases.

During 1989, this nurse noted a marked increase in the demand for *sunna* (around seventy percent of the operations carried out), even though some degree of closure over the urethra was also requested in order to prevent the spraying sound of urination, which is considered "unfeminine." She was also convinced that, in the villages, many colleagues were abandoning the practice of infibulation, which had become more widespread and extreme due to the availability of medical assistants. Some of her colleagues had learned to leave the clitoris intact under the sewn flap of tissue, even if the strength of tradition in some cases thwarted every attempt to attenuate it. According to this nurse, the element most resistant to the abandonment of the practice was the males who insist that it should continue. In Wad Medani, we interviewed a female medical physician who, during the course of her professional activities, tried to convince people, ready to abandon infibulation, to have a "correct *sunna*" performed instead of a clitoridectomy. These subtle acts of persuasion had to be carried out because the communities were strongly resistant to interference with the practice.

To conclude, this physician encountered strong resistance to the abandonment of the practice while carrying out her activity in the rural areas east of the Blue Nile. For this reason, she considers the alternative to infibulation a realistic approach. She consulted a surgeon to develop a suitable surgical technique for the milder *sunna*, but she has not yet determined the best way to implement this alternative.

As far as Somalia is concerned, the information has been drawn from a recent conference, "Advancing in Unity" (October 29-November 2, 2001), held in Hargeisa (Somaliland),[7] and reported in the media as the "Pharaonic Circumcision Conference." The symposium was organized by the London-based Black Women's Health and Family Support Group and was financially supported by Rainb♀ UK, UNICEF-Somalia, and private donors.

Delegates from the United Kingdom, Kenya, Ethiopia, and Sweden participated in the conference. Every Somali region was represented, with the exception of the central and north-eastern regions. The guests — the leaders of the Somali communities who had migrated to Europe — were shocked by the presence of circumcisers and obstetricians among the speakers, openly presenting their professions and practices, ranging from excision to infibulation, as well as re-infibulation. The presentation on re-infibulation, aimed at surgically restoring virginity, both in Somali girls and in immigrant daughters, concentrated on the economic aspects of this practice. Finally, two religious men (*Shaykhs*) presented *sunna* as being a necessary step, thus raising contrasting feelings (ranging from sympathy to bewilderment, and open criticism of the organizers of the symposium). It was of little value to point out that the *hadith* referring to excision is ambiguous, since the participants did not allow themselves to be reassured on this matter. In conclusion, attendees of the symposium agreed that they were against pharaonic circumcision but not against *sunna*. The Somali representatives of immigrants *in diaspora* saw their efforts towards eradicating the practice in Western countries were being frustrated, since the practice persists in their countries of origin.

In 1996, in the Merka district (Lower Shebelli region, Somalia), an alternative ritual celebration to infibulation called "*sunna gudnin*" was proposed and carried out by Mana Abdurahman Ali, who works with the NGO "Water For Life" (WFL). This ritual is a milder version of circumcision (or *sunna*), carried out within the cultural framework of traditional infibulation. The traditional elements of the ceremony, such as the circumcision hut, the ritual dressing of the child and her hair, the presence of relatives, the feasts with friends, the "post-operation" rite carried out with the circumcised girl sitting on the floor, holding her legs out straight and parallel, etc., are retained. The ritual is performed by a *Shaykh* and a health team. It is divided into three distinct stages: the persuasion of the children's mothers, the celebration with the "operation" (*sunna* with clitoris scratching) performed by members of the health team, and later, the visit to the children's houses to verify that the grandmothers, the keepers of the tradition, are in agreement with the ritual.

Sunna gudnin is regularly carried out twice a year, and it has spread to about thirty villages. During its first four years, 1,300 children participated in it. This represents one-third of the schoolgirls of the Merka district. At the end of the year 2000, the project expanded to include 1,080 more girls, on whom the "operation" was gradually reduced to a symbolic micro-lancing.[8]

At present, the program is carried out in six centers, where the girls of all the involved villages gather. The health team includes eleven community health workers who were admitted in progressive order, after having participated in courses organized by the NGO WFL. Furthermore, in two of the centers, Ayuub and Internal Displaced People (IDP), located close to Merka and the headquarters of the NGO, the incidence of clitoral circumcision (*sunna*) as well as the related "micro-scratch" has currently been reduced to zero, as *sunna gudnin* has become a purely symbolic ceremony without any actual cutting.[9]

Our long and well-established relationship of cooperation with the Merka NGO-WFL has permitted us to obtain some videotapes showing the *sunna gudnin* alternative ceremony, carried out from 1996 to 1999. We edited together a videotape using these source materials.

2. VIDEO TAPE UTILIZATION

Recently, we have used the videotape to promote health education among the east African immigrant community living in Italy. Three versions of the video have been prepared — Italian, English, and Somali — and these have been screened for different groups of workers involved in immigration and also for university students.

- The Italian and Somali versions were shown in north-east Italy and, in particular, in Padua, to two presidents of Somali communities, one vice-president of a non-EU Association, and one cultural mediator (all of them Somali). The screening was received coldly and with no apparent interest. Ethnic tensions erupted in the audience because Mana's tribe is considered to occupy a very low status in Somalia. The only person who was enthusiastic about the video was a Somali who belonged to an ethnic group close to Mana's: ("Mana will go to heaven for what she is doing. It has been wise to apply to our population a strategy of taking one step at a time").
- In Turin, the videotape was shown to a Somali head of an NGO legal office for immigrants. The unacceptability of *sunna* in Western countries was recognized. It was also conceded that efforts to eradicate *sunna* in Somalia might succeed because of the presence of a religious team to put the alternative into effect.
- In Florence and Rome, the Italian and Somali language versions were shown to a female gynecologist, a male psychiatrist, and three female cultural mediators (all of them Somali).
- In Rome, the video was strongly attacked because it was judged as being an implausible hoax, performed by actors rather than real

people. The script was defined as being inaccurate with respect to the Somali original. The *sunna* operation was called into question ("Who knows how they performed it?"). Mana's ethnic origin was also a source of criticism.
- In Florence, absolute disagreement was expressed by a cultural mediator responsible for the projects of the American international organization with a great deal of experience in Italy and in Africa.

The English version of the video was presented in the following places:
- In London (1999), it was shown during the "FGM Study Day" to four Somali women: a nurse/obstetrician, a health advisor for social programs, an outreach worker for social and community activities, and a health worker for refugees. They all pinpointed the educational and informational phase as important for the eradication of FGM; only one of them added, talking about *sunna gudnin* in Africa: "If in this way we are able to stop this rubbish, well, it is a positive thing."
- In Ghent (Belgium, 2000), the videotape was shown during the "European Expert Meeting Workshop on FGM" to two university teachers, a "Forward" representative, a Kenyan PhD student, and a Somali representative of a Goteborg-based "Mother Child Program." The Somalis expressed absolute opposition: "This will set us back a decade." Only the Kenyan woman was in favor, recalling the success of alternative programs carried out in her country. An optimistic view was taken by the anthropologist, who underlined the innovative role of religion. The other participants declined to voice their opinions.
- In Sydney (2000), the videotape was presented during the "Sixth International Symposium on Genital Integrity" to all the participants. Here, it was necessary to explain exactly what *sunna* entails. A cultural mediator, representative of the Multicultural Area of the Health Unit of Western Sydney, was not in favor of the alternative. The representatives of the two Australian Somali communities did not voice their opinions.
- In the United States, F. P. Hosken was personally informed of the videotape, but she refused to report the story in her *Hosken News,* because she is against any form of medicalization of the practice and against its financing from outside Somalia.
- In Germany, the videotape was shown to Herta Haas, co-founder of the Hamburg NGO-based "Terres des Femmes." Above all, she admired the courage displayed by Mana. She concluded: "I think that it's always much better to do something!"

The Italian version of the video has been shown in:

- Venice (Ca' Foscari University, Faculty of Literature and Philosophy) to twenty-five students, during a seminar on Cultural Anthropology. Acceptance of the change in the practice — connected to a new religious interpretation — impressed them greatly. The lecturer of anthropology underlined the fact that, in the Koran, female circumcision is not mentioned and that excision is mentioned in the *hadith* only. Other important points captured from the video were: "The lack of attention towards the mothers of the children (attention was given to the grandmothers)," "The absence of the fathers," "The presence of the ancestors, even if dead, as they have a social space — our fathers made a mistake in performing pharaonic circumcision."

- Padua, to about twenty students during the "Postgraduate course on Rural Development for Emerging Countries." These students were struck by the lack of involvement of the male counterpart in the ceremony ("Can't a husband convince his wife at home?"). One doubt was expressed: "What is more important in Merka: the conscience of the grandmothers or the religious clarifications supplied by the *Shaykhs*?" It was viewed as positive that a frontal attack on a pharaonic circumcision was not made in the videotape and that the traditional and religious aspects were safeguarded, therefore, avoiding physical consequences for the girls.

- Padua again, to approximately one-hundred-fifty psychology students at the University of Padua. They asked themselves: "Could it be possible that *sunna*, presented to them as a religious practice, will become as difficult to eradicate in the future, as infibulation is now?" And, as far as immigrants in Italy are concerned, "Shouldn't it be possible to accept them together with their cultural beliefs until they themselves change after more information and education?" "Is it possible for them to be operated on in religious centers?"

- The Italian version, with Arabic translation, was shown to thirty Sudanese students (University of Karthoum) after a seminar on FGM. The nine girls present (all of them infibulated) continued to ask for information on the practice and its consequences on female health, as they were unable to understand the video's presentation of this material. The video captured their attention because of its surgical aspects, and it was considered to be slightly positive." We cannot judge, as we do not exactly know the habits of Somalis. "The male students referred mostly to their compassion for the suffering of the girls. They suggested that, in order to eradicate pharaonic circumcision in their country, more information and education is needed because the practice is still widely performed in rural areas.

Similar to the Somalis of Merka, they reject pharaonic circumcision because this practice is seen as being particular to Egypt and is not a Sudanese tradition. Regarding the choice of a partner, they stated that they are in favor of individual freedom without interference from the families.

3.   DISCUSSION AND CONCLUSION

The present evolution of circumcision, gathered from Sudanese and Somali data, is geared more towards an attenuation of the practice of *sunna* than towards its complete eradication since it is, in fact, the local populations who oppose the latter. *Sunna* appears to find a certain degree of support in the Koran that infibulation does not. In this sense, the role of religious authorities is of great importance, as they are the mediators of change in public opinion.

There is also a great deal of research into technical strategies aimed at reducing the invasive aspect of infibulation (to leave the clitoris intact but hidden under a flap of skin, a closure over the urethra to attenuate the urine flux, etc.), that, at least for Sudan, we have learned from individual operators. *Sunna gudnin* is the only ritually complete and well-organized alternative aimed at changing the practice of infibulation.[10] It appears to be increasing in frequency, even though it is limited geographically. *Sunna gudnin* is systematically carried out twice a year, and dates back almost six years. It has been accepted by about one-third of the female population, and it is gradually evolving into a purely symbolic, non-surgical ritual.

Alternatives of the practice of infibulation appear to be specific to the various populations who devise them. Consequently, they cannot be exported or extended to other communities or applied universally. This has been established by the comments made by the various groups who viewed the *sunna gudnin* videotape. Only in exceptional cases did the alternative *sunna gudnin* ritual presented in the film meet with approval. This came from a Somali belonging to the same ethnic group as Mana, and from Herta Haas.

The Somali highlighted the brilliant but simple logic of the new ritual, whose strengths are the persuasion phase, the *Shaykh* speeches and their efficacy in quoting the *hadiths* of the prophet Mohammed, the intelligent use of metaphors, which is quite fitting for the Somali population, such as the fact that they "play" with imagination, inventing historical backgrounds that are dubious (i.e., the myth of the Pharaoh to explain the origin of infibulation). There are other important aspects too: the choice of persons who are esteemed and respected by the community, the traditional nurse converted to *sunna*, the grandmothers who keep the tradition, in short, the involvement of the whole community.

Herta Haas is against any form of medicalization of the practice, but in a practical way. She believes that, in particular environments, an alternative ritual is necessary, instead of a clear-cut break with traditions, and she refers to many other examples in various African regions. "We must understand that people are not able to completely ban a custom so rooted in their tradition."

In the other cases, the video was criticized and/or regarded with deep concern by Somali viewers. The low status of Mana's ethnic group was emphasized. This fact deterred us from showing the video to Somali women living in Italy. Even the Sudanese, close to Somalis because of their environment, their way of life (pastoral farming), and their circumcision traditions, were able to draw accurate ethnic inferences from the video. This is because the alternative ritual, presently carried out in Africa, is only valid for the groups who devised them. These alternatives cannot be exported and used for the same populations *in diaspora*, whose tendency is to faithfully reproduce and cling to all of the ethnic traditions of their homelands.

As far as the Western viewers are concerned, the videotape became the object of interesting observations. Because the reality of genital cutting is too complex and far removed from our cultural experience, Western viewers focused only on the bloody, surgical aspects of the rituals presented in the video and passed conventional judgments.

In conclusion, we underscore the fact that we do not want to propose ourselves as supporters and promoters of the medicalization of the practice of *sunna*. Instead, we report the evolution that infibulation is at present experiencing in East Africa. Nowadays, *sunna gudnin* represents one of the forms of genital cutting in Africa that, we hope, will eventually lead to the complete eradication of all forms of genital cutting.

Of course, we cannot conceal the danger that, if the replacement of infibulation by *sunna* is seen as an improvement in female health conditions, it is possible that it could become socially entrenched and reinforced by adherence to Islamic law. Nevertheless, we agree with a Somali social worker interviewed in London: "Circumcised women will stop circumcising their daughters thanks to education. I was infibulated, but my daughter is not. She underwent *sunna*, but she will not perform *sunna* on her daughter."[11] This is how the practice will stop, and is exactly what the first author of this paper predicted in 1986 when she examined the problem.[12]

The same opinion is expressed by Ellen Gruenbaum for Sudan: "Where there is infibulation, the result of a process of change might be to modify, rather than to eliminate, female genital cutting. Certainly it would be easier to mobilize Sudanese families towards that change rather than reject all forms immediately."[13]

Pia Grassivaro Gallo et al.

REFERENCES

1. Grassivaro Gallo P, Rabuffetti L, Viviani F. Sunna gudnin. An alternative ritual to infibulation in Merka Somalia. In: Denniston G.C., Hodges F.M., Milos M.F. Understanding circumcision. A multi-disciplinary approach to a Multi-Dimensional Problem. New York: Kluwer Academic/Plenum Publishers, 2001. pp. 99-111.
2. Hassan AR Amna. Resumé de l'impact de la récherche sur les "Les MGF Consequences psychosociales et sexuelles et changement d'attitudes dans Khartoum Nord et Nile Est". Bull. du Comité Inter-africain, no. 28, (December 5-7, 2000).
3. Hassan AR Amna. FGM Historical Background, Views in Islamic Shari'a et Recent Research's Findings on MGF, 2001, in press.
4. Sanderson LP. The Babiker Bedri Scientific Association for Women's Studies Workshops for the Abolition of all Forms of Female Genital Mutilation in the Sudan. Notes and Records. 1982. pp. 65-72.
5. Nagla Dawelbact, personal communication, 2001.
6. Gruenbaum E. The female circumcision controversy: An anthropological perspective. Philadelphia: University of Pennsylvania Press, 2000.
7. Jamila Said Musse, personal communication, 2001.
8. Grassivaro Gallo P, Rabuffetti L, Viviani F. Sunna gudnin. An alternative ritual to infibulation in Merka Somalia. In: Denniston G.C., Hodges F.M., Milos M.F. Understanding circumcision. A multi-disciplinary approach to a Multi-Dimensional Problem. New York: Kluwer Academic/Plenum Publishers, 2001. pp. 99-111.
9. Mana Abdurahman Ali and E. Sommaville, personal communication, April-May 2002.
10. Grassivaro Gallo P, Rabuffetti L, Viviani F. Sunna gudnin. An alternative ritual to infibulation in Merka Somalia. In: Denniston G.C., Hodges F.M., Milos M.F. Understanding circumcision. A multi-disciplinary approach to a Multi-Dimensional Problem. New York: Kluwer Academic/Plenum Publishers, 2001. pp. 99-111.
11. Faduma Hassan, personal communication, 1999.
12. Grassivaro Gallo P. La Circoncisione Femminile in Somalia: Una Ricerca Sul Campo. Milan: Franco Angeli, 1986. pp. 57, 155.
13. Gruenbaum E. The female circumcision controversy: An anthropological perspective. Philadelphia: University of Pennsylvania Press, 2000. p. 195.

Chapter 12

"SOMETHING LESS THAN JOYFUL"
Jewish Americans and the Circumcision Dilemma

Leonard B. Glick, Ph.D., MD
Hampshire College

Abstract: Contemporary Jewish Americans are not a monolithic population; to the contrary, they are very diverse in religious beliefs and affiliations. Nevertheless, most seem to take for granted that their infant sons should be circumcised. With only the vaguest understanding of the traditional liturgy, and content to accept claims for medical or "hygienic" benefits, many choose circumcision by a physician for their infant sons, and have little or no interest in religious prescriptions. Even most of those who accept ritual circumcision have very little understanding of what happens or why. Although many circumcision liturgies have been extensively modified and "sanitized" nowadays, the traditional liturgy includes three features that might cause considerable unease if understood: biblical passages referring to wallowing in blood, human sacrifice, and a "peace pact" following a double murder. This paper explains the significance of the passages in their ritual context, then describes how authors of contemporary books addressed to mainstream audiences try to construct acceptable interpretations of the passages and justifications for continuation of the rite. Most Jewish Americans now say that they observe only those ritual practices (if any) that contribute to their "spiritual" welfare. If and when hospitals discontinue "routine" circumcisions, Jewish-American parents will need to decide whether to accept a ritual procedure that is so obviously inappropriate for life in contemporary America.

Key words: Circumcision, Judaism, Jews

1.   INTRODUCTION

In a widely read book entitled *American Judaism,* first published in 1957, the sociologist Nathan Glazer commented on what he called an "interesting anomaly" in the ritual practices of Reform Jews — supposedly the most

Flesh and Blood, Edited by Denniston et al.
Kluwer Academic/Plenum Publishers, New York 2004

acculturated Jewish Americans: "If one is interested in modernizing the Jewish religion, in bringing it into conformity with enlightened and progressive views, in abandoning any rite that does not serve to ennoble and uplift, the logical place to begin, one would think, is with circumcision." For a time some Reform Jews even tried to eliminate such an "innocent and even edifying" ceremony as *bar mitzvah*, he continued; yet "circumcision remained." He repeated the statement in the book's second edition, which appeared in 1972.[1]

Now, thirty years later, Glazer's observation seems equally or even more pertinent. For the fact is that, despite their progressive leanings on many issues, most Jewish Americans still seem to favor circumcision — a custom vaguely understood, if at all, but for the most part not even questioned. Moreover, their self-designated "representatives," functionaries in Jewish-American organizations, are likely to condemn any hint of opposition or critical examination. So it is understandable that in the view of those hoping to end circumcision in America, the most prominent defenders of the practice — those likely to stand in the way of every move in the desired direction — are thought to be "the Jews." This is seldom stated openly, of course, because of the unwelcome prospect of being labeled "anti-Semite" (or, in the case of Jewish critics, "self-hating Jew"). I suggest, though, that it would be helpful to seek more complete understanding of this population, seemingly so intransigent on this single point, so primordially "stubborn." Considered categorically (which is precisely what I shall discourage), they can indeed seem puzzling: largely well educated and prosperous, yet determined (so it appears) to defend an anachronistic practice that inflicts pain and harm on helpless infants. Viewed through the lens of modern sociology, however, most Jewish Americans turn out to be already well distanced from the kind of mentality that undergirds unquestioning acceptance of circumcision — so much so that it seems very possible that Jewish support for the practice may begin to melt away when American hospitals discontinue their ill-considered policy of promoting "routine" circumcisions.

What do we know about contemporary Jewish Americans, and how might that matter in the future? First, depending partly on who is and is not counted, the "core" Jewish population totals about five and a half million, only about 2.2% of the American population. Second, when it comes to religious observance and ethnic self-identification, Jewish Americans are considerably more diverse than other Americans may suppose. To the degree that the diversity is recognized, it is usually understood and described in language familiar to Christians: just as there are Baptists, Presbyterians, Roman Catholics, and the rest, so among Jews there are Orthodox, Conservative, and Reform. More knowledgeable commentators may add the rather inscrutable Hasidim, and, at the other end of the spectrum, the seldom mentioned progressives called Reconstructionists.[2] But the fact is that denominational categorization, although useful to a degree, not only fails to describe the contemporary Jewish-American population completely enough but distorts its actual composition by blurring distinctions that matter most.

Over the last two decades or so, a number of sociologists have published revealing studies that provide a much more complete portrait of Jewish Americans than emerges when one is limited to such denominational terms as Orthodox, Conservative, and Reform. Their most significant single finding is that the overall trend is clearly away from religious orthodoxy and ethnic particularism, toward assertion of "American" as primary identity. To state this somewhat differently, most perceive themselves as Jewish Americans, not as American Jews.[3] The distinction matters. It is common knowledge that "Jewish" is both a religious and an ethnic label; a convert to Judaism becomes a Jew. But ever since the onset of modernity, with its emphasis on individualism and personal choice, it has been possible to separate the two identities — specifically, to maintain ethnic Jewish identification without necessarily accepting any of the beliefs or practices associated with the religion called Judaism. (For that matter, it has also been possible to try to abandon both forms of identification, although I think it is generally recognized that ethnicity often proves more tenacious.) Thus, as many Jewish Americans see it, parallel populations to their own are not Protestants, Catholics, and the like, but Italian Americans, African Americans, and so on. Most beliefs and customs connected with religious particularism — "chosen people" ideology (long discarded by most), dietary regulations, rigorous endogamy, residential separatism, etc. — are now far less operative.

It has become evident also that the truly salient divide in the contemporary Jewish-American population is not between named denominations but between, on the one hand, those who are intent on preserving religious orthodoxy and unwavering ethnic particularism and, on the other, those who believe that Jewish identity is most meaningfully expressed, not through acceptance of dogma or adherence to formal ritual practices, but through commitment to social justice (a favorite term) and to such ideals as liberalism, philanthropy, and personal responsibility. Of the two populations, the latter is by far the larger; an estimate of about 85% of the total seems in line with the results of most recent studies. This large group is itself divisible, however, although again not into the familiar denominational categories; rather, one finds several substantial subgroups differing in degrees of involvement in Jewish concerns. First are those usually characterized as "moderates" or "moderately affiliated." They are an influential component, largely middle-aged or older; I'll say more about them in a moment. Second is another sizable group, more heavily concentrated in the under-forty population, who readily acknowledge Jewish ethnic identity but express little or no interest in formal religious concerns, and participate only minimally, if at all, in explicitly Jewish activities of any kind. Finally, another significant segment, now estimated at a million or more, and again concentrated in the younger age cohort, has abandoned identification with Judaism and Jewishness so completely as to have virtually disappeared from the Jewish-American sociological screen.[4]

A recent study by two prominent research scholars is especially revealing with regard to the "moderately affiliated" population. *The Jew Within*, by Steven M. Cohen and Arnold M. Eisen, reports on responses by a large sample of middle-aged Jewish Americans, self-identified as moderately committed to Judaism and Jewish ethnicity, to questions about their religious beliefs and personal practices.[5] Their foremost conclusion is that their subjects are intensely, one might say passionately, individualistic. In obvious contrast to what would be expected from Orthodox respondents, these middle-of-the-roaders presented themselves as "universalist, liberal, and personalist." They declared that they themselves decided "which rituals they will observe and how they will observe them...which beliefs they will hold, which loyalties they will acknowledge." They stated that they did not believe "in special divine commandments to the Jews, or special divine providence watching over Jews."[6] So, despite their firmly held Jewish identity, they are liberal modern Americans professing values more consistent with multiculturalism than with ethnic particularism.

What did Cohen and Eisen discover about the attitudes of their subjects to circumcision? Unfortunately, nothing, since their extensive questionnaire did not include even a single question about what would seem to have been an obvious topic for their project.[7] But we're free to draw our own conclusions. If even the more conservatively inclined in the non-Orthodox segment are making their own decisions about ritual observances, what should one conclude about the much larger number — mostly younger, therefore more likely to have parenthood still ahead — who are minimally attached to Jewish observance or entirely disaffiliated? As for circumcision, it seems reasonable to assume that if most Jewish Americans still accept the practice, this is not because they are Jewish but because they are Americans.

With this much said, however, it must be acknowledged that many individuals in the "moderately affiliated" category still seem determined to hold on to circumcision, come what may. It is unfortunate that the questions one would most like to have answered — for example, how many would insist on circumcision if physicians recommended against it — have not been asked.[8] I think it is safe to say, though, that for the majority of the moderately affiliated — most of whom, it might be noted, have no clear idea of how many Gentile infants are being circumcised — the image of circumcision as a singular Jewish custom is so deep-rooted, so entrenched, that even questioning its appropriateness raises eyebrows. To put it differently, they believe that since Jews have always circumcised their infant sons, they always will — and they know nothing to challenge that conviction.

Would this attitude endure if more Jewish Americans knew something about the actual meaning of ritual circumcision? In particular, what would be the response of that large and steadily growing category of minimally engaged young adults who are now becoming parents? Are they likely to fall dutifully in line, taking circumcision for granted? For the present, many new parents adopt the least problematic path. They accept claims for the procedure's medical or "hygienic" benefits and simply agree to the circumcision recommended in many hospitals, enabling them to fit comfortably into the American mainstream without having to ask such perplexing questions as how infant genital surgery contributes to Jewish "survival."

Those wanting to preserve more sense of specifically Jewish significance for the procedure have been turning to the recently constituted cohort of "physician-mohels," trained by representatives of the Reform and Conservative denominations, who perform reassuringly professional foreskin removal in the home, accompanied by tailored liturgy and religious homilies designed to provide an appropriately "spiritual" setting for the surgery. Even in those instances, however, very few family members and witnesses at a ritual circumcision have more than the vaguest notions of what is happening or why. The usual word for the rite is *Brit* (or, in the more traditional Ashkenazic pronunciation, *Bris*), meaning "Covenant." The complete term, seldom used in speech, is *Brit Milah*, "Covenant of Circumcision." It can be said with certainty that, aside from the Orthodox minority, very few Jewish Americans are now able to explain what the phrase really means. The myth of Abraham's covenant, "sealed" by his auto-circumcision, is about as familiar as a tale from the *Ramayana*.[9]

All rabbis, ranging from Orthodox to Reform, agree that a circumcision without ritual — that is, without recitation of a liturgy — has no religious validity. Although this is doctrinally correct, the fact is that many young Jewish-American parents either don't realize it or don't care. Since the customary notion is that a circumcision of any kind "makes the boy Jewish," surgery performed by a hospital physician often seems preferable to a ritual procedure performed by a mohel with unknown qualifications — and, in any event, requires nothing on the parents' part: no participation in a puzzling rite, no need to witness the surgery, no celebration with invited guests. Performed out of sight, the matter is soon out of mind (at least for whichever parent avoids the task of diaper changing).

Nowadays, most Jewish Americans, particularly those under forty, have little or no knowledge of Hebrew and only limited understanding of even the most familiar Jewish rituals. When it comes to the ritual circumcision liturgy, knowledge and understanding are near zero. That may be just as well, though, for defenders of the practice, since the liturgy in its original form would surely not attract the individualistic "moderate" Jews interviewed by Cohen and Eisen, let alone the large number who are peripheral or non-committed. The liturgy has already been heavily revised in efforts to accord with contemporary sensibilities. Even moderate ("Modern") Orthodox Jews have introduced some changes, and Reform Jews have gone even further still. But it is the distasteful passages that are the least incidental or dispensable; in fact, they are central to the rite's meaning and intention.

I'll try to explain this by describing the rite and focusing on several liturgical passages. One refers to a "peace pact" between God and Israel following a double murder. Another encourages the infant to live on, though it is "wallowing" in its own blood. Two others, phrased in oblique language, seem to call for acceptance of the sacrificed foreskin as redemption for the child, perhaps as a substitute for sacrifice of the child himself. By radically revising the liturgy to eliminate passages of this sort, the rite, with its genital surgery, has been preserved by concealing its actual meaning. What, then, was and is the true purpose and intent of a ritual circumcision?

2.   REVEALING THE CONCEALED: THE MEANING OF THE RITE

The overarching message in a ritual circumcision is that Jewish men must declare publicly their acceptance of sexual restraint, religious compliance, and unwavering loyalty to the male Jewish collective. In Lawrence Hoffman's words, the rite is "a ceremonial celebration of the obligation that binds men to each other in rabbinic culture."[10] It is not the infant who declares acceptance and loyalty, of course, but his father, who announces at the very beginning of the rite that he is "ready and prepared to perform the commandment." It might be said, then, that the rite requires the father to submit his son to circumcision as a public declaration of his own submission to the ethnic collective.[11] Nor does the rite "make the child Jewish" as is commonly supposed, since only birth to a Jewish mother accomplishes that; rather, it affirms the father's commitment to ensuring that the child will follow in his path.

Embedded within the rite are messages recalling an ancient past about which most Jewish fathers know little or nothing. The biblical quotations forming the core of the rite are, like nearly all such texts, subject to almost endless interpretation. Nevertheless, I shall try to show that, considered together, they present an unmistakable command: that fathers must offer their sons as atonement for the sinful sexual nature that plagues all men, and as public affirmation of their own loyalty, and, in the future, that of their sons, to the male-centered Jewish community.[12]

Since versions of the liturgy adopted by various constituencies differ substantially, I'll present a composite version, based on that in Lawrence Hoffman's study of ritual circumcision, *Covenant of Blood*, which cites two mainstream Orthodox liturgies (which I have also consulted), and *Bris Milah*, a manual by Paysach Krohn issued by a prominent ultra-Orthodox publisher.[13] Hoffman is a Reform rabbi and scholar, a specialist in the history of liturgy. The Krohn manual is especially instructive, since it presents an unabridged version of the traditional rite. Translations of biblical texts will be based mainly on the Jewish Publication Society edition, with alternatives added where appropriate.[14] First I'll present a comprehensive version (without comment) incorporating all elements that will be of particular interest, and omitting nothing that could be considered integral or essential. (Sequences differ somewhat in various liturgies, but this has no particular bearing on our discussion.) Then I'll discuss the sections that tell us most about the central message of the rite, some or even most of which have been ignored or eliminated in contemporary versions.

I have placed reference numbers immediately *following* sections of the liturgy to be analyzed.

2.1 The Liturgy

As the infant is brought into the room where he is to be circumcised, the assembled witnesses exclaim in welcome, "Blessed is he who comes." The mohel takes the infant, perhaps displays him to the group, and recites a brief invocation recalling the opening verse of Genesis 17, in which the Lord appears to Abram just before issuing the command that he circumcise himself:

> "[T]he Holy One, Blessed be He, said to Abraham, our father, 'Walk in My ways and be blameless' [or 'Walk before Me and be perfect']." [1]

Then he recites a passage from Chapter 25 of Numbers:

> The Lord spoke to Moses, saying, "Phinehas, son of Eleazar son of Aaron the priest, has turned back My wrath from the Israelites by displaying among them his passion for Me, so that I did not wipe out the Israelite people in My passion. Say, therefore, 'I grant him My pact of friendship' [or 'My covenant of peace']."[15] [2]

The mohel then places the child either on a chair designated as "the chair of Elijah," or on the knees of the man, called *sandek*, who will hold him during the circumcision; or the *sandek* may himself sit in Elijah's chair.[16]

The mohel says, "This is the chair of Elijah the prophet, remembered for good." The mohel and the father declare that they are "ready and willing" to perform the commandment. [3]

As the mohel circumcises the infant, or immediately thereafter, the father blesses the Lord, "who has commanded us to bring him into the covenant of Abraham, our father." The assembled witnesses proclaim, "As he has entered the covenant, so may he enter Torah, marriage [literally, the wedding canopy], and good deeds."

Now the mohel blesses a cup of wine and delivers the following invocation:

> Blessed art Thou, Lord, our God, King of the universe, who sanctified the beloved one from the womb, and placed Your statute in his flesh, and sealed his descendants with the sign of the holy covenant. Therefore, as reward for this, O Living God, our Portion and our Rock, may You command that the beloved of our flesh be delivered from the pit, for the sake of His covenant that He has placed in our flesh. Blessed art thou, Lord, who creates [literally, cuts] the covenant.[17] [4]

Then he places a drop or two of the wine on the infant's lips and recites a prayer announcing the child's name and calling yet again, and in still more explicit language, for his deliverance or salvation:

> Our God and God of our fathers, preserve (or sustain) this child for his father and mother, and let his name in Israel be [name], son of [father's name]. May the father rejoice in the issue from his loins, and may the mother receive happiness from the fruit of her womb, as it is written: "When I passed by you and saw you wallowing in your blood, I said to you, 'Live in spite of your blood.' Yea, I said to you, 'Live in spite of your blood' [alternatively, and more precisely: 'In your blood, live']." [5]

This prayer continues with reference to the covenant and to the circumcision of Isaac, and concludes with another call for the child to enter Torah study, marriage, and good deeds. Now the mohel recites another prayer suggestive of redemptive sacrifice:

> Master of the universe, may it be Your will to regard and accept this as though I had offered him before Your glorious throne. In Your abundant mercy, send through Your holy angels a holy and pure soul to [child's name, son of father's name], who has just been circumcised to Your great name. May his heart, opened as wide as the entrance to the Temple, be open to Your holy Torah, to learn and to teach, to observe and to perform. [6]

He follows this with a prayer asking that the "tender child" be granted "complete healing," and that his father be deemed worthy of raising him to Torah, marriage, and good deeds. Everyone says, "Amen."

The rite ends with a standard concluding prayer (*Alenu*, declaring acceptance of God's will that the people of Israel be different from other nations). Then everyone adjourns for a festive meal.

Each number in brackets in the next section refers to the corresponding number in the liturgy.

2.2 Interpreting the Liturgy

[1] In the first verse of Genesis 17, the Lord announces himself to Abram by an unusual name, Shaddai, and orders him to "walk before me and be *tamim*." Most often as used in the Torah the word means flawless, perfectly formed, without blemish. Rabbinic commentators have adopted this line of interpretation throughout the centuries, the argument being that the foreskin is a physical imperfection — a "blemish" — that must be removed to create perfect men.[18] In this particular context, however, the Jewish Publication Society translation — using the word "blameless" — has much to recommend it. Although in biblical usage *tamim* usually refers to *physical* perfection in animals, it may also carry the meaning of perfection of *character*, which seems precisely what the translators understood here. Interpreting the word in physical terms accords conveniently with the rabbinic doctrine that the foreskin is a physical imperfection; but it seems more plausible that its original meaning in this passage had to do with "blameless" character and behavior, not with the need to remove a physical "blemish."

[2] The entire passage about Phinehas has been eliminated from most liturgies, although Krohn's Orthodox manual retains it (translating the concluding phrase, *briti shalom*, accurately as "My covenant of Peace").[19] Considered in isolation, these verses are so enigmatic that surely all but the most well-informed readers or listeners would be hard put to explain how they apply to infant circumcision. The matter becomes somewhat clearer, though, when we read the biblical story. While the Israelites were encamped in Moabite territory, the final stop on their journey into Canaan, Israelite men "profaned themselves by whoring with the Moabite women" and participating in sacrifices to the Moabite deity, Baal-peor. The "incensed" Israelite God imposed a plague on the entire community and commanded Moses to have the leading transgressors "publicly impaled." But before Moses could carry out the executions, Aaron's grandson Phinehas entered a tent where a high-ranking Israelite man was copulating with an equally high-ranking Midianite (not Moabite) woman and drove a spear through them both. This deed so gratified the Lord that he relented and ended the plague (although twenty-four thousand had already died). The liturgy's quoted passage on turning back wrath follows. The Lord was still so angry, though,

that he instructed Moses to attack and defeat the Midianites as punishment for "the trickery they practiced against you."[20]

The Krohn manual explains that Phinehas was rewarded for risking his life "to avenge the desecration of God's name."[21] This "desecration" was not worship of an alien deity, however, since Phinehas's deed had nothing to do with that; the "desecration" was insertion of a circumcised penis into forbidden territory. According to kabbalistic doctrine, circumcision consecrates the Jewish phallus by inscribing on it *Shaddai*, the name by which God identified himself to Abram in Genesis 17, just before instructing him to circumcise himself; hence, adulterous intercourse or any intercourse with a non-Israelite woman violates the sanctity of the consecrated organ.[22] In a larger sense, the Phinehas passage opens the liturgy as a warning against any form of sexual misbehavior.

[3] Although Elijah's presence at the rite is customarily explained by reference to his traditional identification as the "herald" of the Messiah, or by describing him as a "protector" of children, there is good reason to conclude that in this context he is not an entirely benign figure. An article by Lifsa Schachter points out that Phinehas and Elijah are closely associated as men who "saved the Israelites from the consequences of their sins," but also as "agents of punishment, bringing death to individuals who had sinned." They are invoked, Schachter suggests, "to avert the disaster which the sins of licentiousness and idolatry bring in their wake."[23] The reference here is to an episode recorded in Chapter 19 of I Kings. Elijah has just defeated, then slaughtered, the "prophets of Baal" (I Kings 18:21-40). When the furious Jezebel threatens to kill him in retaliation, he flees for his life and, following a journey of forty days and forty nights (sustained by a single meal of bread and water), he arrives at "the mountain of God at Horeb" and enters a cave to sleep. The Lord appears and asks:

'Why are you here, Elijah?' He replied, 'I am moved by zeal for the Lord, the God of Hosts, for the Israelites have forsaken Your covenant, torn down Your altars, and put Your prophets to the sword. I alone am left, and they are out to take my life.' (I Kings 19:9-10)[24]

Later in the same chapter the Lord assures Elijah that he will see to it that only seven thousand Israelites — "every knee that has not knelt to Baal and every mouth that has not kissed him" — will survive his wrath (I Kings 19:18).

Note that the crime of the wayward Israelites was having "forsaken" the Lord's covenant — presumably a reference to the covenant at Sinai but obviously reverberating in this context with Abraham's earlier covenant. In any event, as Schachter observes, the essential message is unmistakable: Any violation of the "covenant" is the ultimate sin.

Schachter also points out that the references to "Torah, marriage, and good deeds" are not just platitudes; they are "actually the obverse" of the threat of punishment expressed in the references to Phinehas and Elijah. The prayer can be interpreted as a call for religious observance ("Torah") "*as against idolatry*," marriage "*as against sexual licentiousness*," and proper behavior ("good deeds").[25]

[4] Although the sanctified "beloved one" may appear to be the infant being circumcised, Hoffman interprets the prayer to say that God set the original "statute" in Abraham's flesh, and thereby sealed (Hoffman says "stamped") his descendants with the sign of the covenant. Hence, "the beloved one" is Abraham, who "becomes the model for all Jewish fathers."[26] But the "beloved of our flesh" is the infant. Hoffman also explains that in rabbinic texts "the pit" is a reference to *She'ol*, the biblical term for an underworld where the dead live an eternal featureless existence.[27] The prayer asks that the infant be "delivered from the pit," that is, from death, as a reward for his father's having sacrificed his foreskin.[28]

To carry this a short step further: Since circumcision is obviously a kind of sacrifice, or a representation of sacrifice, might infant circumcision have been adopted as a substitution or replacement for child sacrifice? The fact is that child sacrifice was widely practiced in ancient Palestine, and there is no good reason to assume that the Israelites differed in this regard from their Canaanite neighbors. The Hebrew Scriptures provide two kinds of evidence. First, a passage in Exodus (22:28) has Yahweh speaking quite plainly: "You shall give Me the first-born among your sons." In his exhaustive study of this subject, Jon D. Levenson shows that, despite efforts of some interpreters to find other meanings here, "give" means just what it suggests.[29] Moreover, in two other chapters in Exodus (13:1-2, 11-15; 34:19-20) we find the Lord demanding that first-born sons, along with various first-born animals, be "redeemed." Of course, the redemption theme appears also in the most familiar of all child-sacrifice tales, the near-sacrifice of Isaac (Genesis 22). That event has also been interpreted away (the argument being that the Lord offered a ram substitute to indicate his disapproval of child sacrifice); but, as Levenson remarks, "it is passing strange to condemn child sacrifice through a narrative in which a father is richly rewarded for his willingness to carry out that very practice....Abraham will have his multitude of descendants only because he was willing to sacrifice the son who is destined to beget them."[30] We might note also the rather obvious point that Abraham was ordered to sacrifice the son whose birth was the reward for his earlier sacrifice, his auto-circumcision.

As for the second kind of evidence, the Scriptures are revealingly endowed with references to worship of Molech, the most fearful and repulsive of alien deities, the god to whom infants and small children (girls and boys) were sacrificed, probably in numbers one would rather not imagine.[31] Molech was a Canaanite underworld deity whose sacrificial site was at Tophet, or Topheth, ("oven," "furnace"), in the Valley of Hinnom, near Jerusalem.[32] Without equating sacrifices to the two deities, Molech and Yahweh, Levenson concludes that Yahweh-worship also involved child sacrifice.[33]

If child sacrifice did indeed exist, it was probably eliminated from Israelite religion by about the sixth century BCE. In the book of the prophet Jeremiah, active in the years just before and after 600 BCE, we find Yahweh not only condemning child sacrifice but denying that he ever favored such a practice:

> For the people of Judah have done what displeases Me...they have built the shrines of Topheth in the Valley of Ben-hinnom to burn their sons and daughters in fire — which I never commanded, which never came to My mind....They have built shrines to Baal, to put their children to the fire as burnt offerings to Baal — which I never commanded, never decreed, and which never came to My mind.[34]

Levenson suggests that the Israelites appear to have adopted a number of "substitution rituals" for literal sacrifice of first-born sons, most notably the paschal lamb of the Exodus legend, whose blood redeemed Israelite children while those of the Egyptians were being slaughtered. But how about circumcision? Was this too a "sublimation" of child sacrifice? As we'll note shortly, ritual circumcision *requires* shedding of blood — hard to interpret other than as symbolic blood sacrifice. Although we cannot be certain, Levenson concludes, the evidence suggests that "the impulse to sacrifice the first-born son remained potent long after the literal practice had become odious and fallen into desuetude."[35] We can interpret the prayer, therefore, as offering thanks that the child's circumcision redeems him from sacrifice.

[5] Immediately after reciting the passage referring to "wallowing" in blood, the mohel dips his finger into a cup of wine and places a drop on the infant's lips. It is often claimed that the wine is administered to distract and calm the child; but, as we'll see in a moment, there is more to it than that. The passage is drawn from Chapter 16 of Ezekiel. In the original text, the Lord, speaking through Ezekiel, castigates the Israelites for practicing "abominations" and reminds them of how much he has done on their behalf. He addresses the people metaphorically, portraying them as a helpless infant — specifically, a female infant "from the land of the Canaanites," child of a Hittite father and an Amorite mother:

> As for your birth, when you were born your navel cord was not cut, and you were not bathed in water to smooth you; you were not rubbed with salt, nor were you swaddled. No one pitied you enough to do any one of these things for you out of compassion for you; on the day you were born, you were left lying,

rejected, in the open field. When I passed by you and saw you wallowing in your blood, I said to you: "Live in spite of your blood." Yea, I said to you: "Live in spite of your blood." I let you grow like the plants of the field; and you continued to grow up until you attained to womanhood, until your breasts became firm and your hair sprouted.

You were still naked and bare when I passed by you [again] and saw that your time for love had arrived. So I spread My robe over you and covered your nakedness, and I entered into a covenant with you by oath — declares the Lord God; thus you became Mine. I bathed you in water, and washed the blood off you, and anointed you with oil....Your beauty won you fame among the nations, for it was perfected through the splendor which I set upon you — declares the Lord God.[36]

The passage seems to refer to a practice common in biblical times. Unwanted infants, female infants in particular, and especially those that were illegitimate, were abandoned to die from exposure and starvation. Here we read of an abandoned female infant who is rescued, reared to maturity, and "entered" into a covenant. But had it just been "covenant" that attracted the rabbis who designed the liturgy, they could have chosen any of a number of more appropriate passages; what drew them to these verses was the mention of blood. The Jewish Publication Society translation of the key sentence, "Live in spite of your blood," appears to reverse (and perhaps disguise) the literal Hebrew meaning, "In your blood, live." Invocation of this passage in the liturgy seems to say that the blood shed in circumcision brings the reward of life for the infant; it is redemptive.

One of the most explicit expressions of the redemptive blood theme is found in a rabbinic text called *Chapters of Rabbi Eliezer*, composed at various times during or before the ninth century. As this volume tells the Genesis 17 story, Abraham circumcised himself on Yom Kippur, the Day of Atonement. (The reasoning is too labyrinthine for discussion here.) That leads to a discourse on blood as atonement and salvation: "Every year the Holy One, Blessed be He, sees the blood of our father Abraham's circumcision, and He forgives all the sins of Israel."[37]

Further along in this text we encounter another interpretation, frequently cited in rabbinic literature: the blood of circumcision enhances the paschal blood of the Exodus legend:

The Israelites took the blood of the covenant of circumcision, and they put (it) upon the lintel of their houses, and when the Holy One, blessed be He, passed over to plague the Egyptians, He saw the blood of the covenant of circumcision upon the lintel of their houses and the blood of the Paschal lamb. He was filled with compassion on Israel, as it is said, 'And when I passed by thee, and saw thee weltering in thy (twofold) blood, I said unto thee, In thy (twofold) blood,

live; yea, I said unto thee, In thy (twofold) blood, live' (Ezek. 16:6). 'In thy
blood' is not written here, but in 'thy (twofold) blood,' with twofold blood, the
blood of the covenant of circumcision and the blood of the Paschal
lamb....Rabbi Eliezer said: Why did the text say twice, 'I said unto thee, In thy
blood, live; yea, I said unto thee, In thy blood, live'? But the Holy One, blessed
be He, said: By the merit of the blood of the covenant of circumcision and the
blood of the Paschal lamb ye shall be redeemed from Egypt.[38]

Hoffman points out that, whereas God's central promise to Abraham in
Genesis 17 is immense reproductive success ("I will make you exceedingly
fertile" Gen. 17:6), the rabbis chose to emphasize the covenant theme,
replacing the fertility symbolism with "blood as a symbol of
salvation....[T]he blood of the paschal lamb and the blood of circumcision
become merged because both are items given by God specifically to effect
salvation."[39] He points also to another feature of blood symbolism: the
unusual role of wine. In the course of the rite the mohel blesses a cup of
wine but does not sip it — a clear departure from customary practice. He
does place a drop of wine on the child's lips, though, immediately after the
"wallowing" in blood recitation. The blessing over wine is ordinarily recited
by those who intend to drink it, but in this case it is only the infant who
"drinks." Now, says Hoffman, we see why the mohel doesn't sip the wine,
and why no blessing is recited over the wine before it is placed in the
infant's mouth: "It was not meant to be consumed *as wine* at all, but was
instead reserved as an oral transfusion of wine *as blood* for the child. In a
nutshell, blood escapes the system; wine as blood enters it."[40]

[6] Finally, the prayer offering the child before the Lord's "glorious
throne" is additional confirmation that circumcision is interpretable as a
sacrificial offering by the infant's father, in the hope and anticipation that the
child will be found acceptable for redemption and a full life. A part has been
sacrificed to salvage the whole.

This by no means exhausts the possible interpretations, many quite
convincing, that have been offered for this complex rite. In addition to
Hoffman's book, from which I have skimmed only a few of the most notable
points, there is the work of Howard Eilberg-Schwartz, whose book, *The
Savage in Judaism*, includes a luminous chapter on foreskin symbolism and
the significance of "pruning" imagery.[41] My central purpose, however, is not
to offer a comprehensive interpretation of circumcision but to show that the
rite is weighted with meanings, some quite sinister, that most Jewish
Americans nowadays neither know about nor would care to know about.[42]

We have seen, then, that in a ritual circumcision the child's father offers
his son's foreskin as a bloody sacrifice, perhaps as a replacement for what
may once have been sacrifice of the entire child. He declares
acknowledgment of paternity, readiness to submit the child to a perilous

procedure, avowal of sexual restraint in the child's future, and intention to raise him as a loyal member of the male-centered collective.[43] In effect, he represses expression of his own reluctance and dread, surrendering himself and his son to the will of male elders.

I should emphasize again that although everything I have described is an integral part of the traditional circumcision liturgy, the distasteful features are often eliminated, even by those now called "modern Orthodox." Recently I spoke with a very active physician-mohel, certified by the Reform *Berit Mila* Board (their spelling), who developed his version of the service with the Orthodox Krohn manual as his principal reference — so he could not have missed the texts I've been discussing. When I asked him about Phinehas, the pit of destruction, and wallowing in blood, he appeared puzzled, then assured me that there was nothing of that sort in *his* service. His wife expressed obvious surprise and repugnance. (Even though it was she who had encouraged her husband to undertake the role of mohel, she remarked later that if any cutting had to be performed on infant girls, she wouldn't want to be Jewish.)[44]

3.   UNANSWERABLE QUESTIONS, QUESTIONABLE ANSWERS

Prospective parents seeking information about ritual circumcision are likely to turn to popular books on Jewish ritual practices. What do they learn about the circumcision liturgy, and what conclusions might they draw with regard to the meaning and purpose of the rite?

Although most books addressed to Jewish parents adopt the cheerful, non-critical perspective characteristic of American advice literature, authors seem well aware of the apprehension and dread surrounding circumcision. Probably the most widely read writer in this genre is Anita Diamant, whose *Jewish Baby Book* acknowledges even in the preface the anxiety of parents who feel "dazed, out of control, and something less than joyful" when faced with the prospect of having their infant sons circumcised. Since Diamant characterizes her book as a description of "liberal Jewish practice in America," meaning "all non-Orthodox movements," she must assume that her readers require something more convincing than unqualified statements about divine demands. Her task is to justify the ways of Judaism to apprehensive parents seeking rational explanation and reassurance.[45]

Diamant begins with admission of her own discomfort. She explains that while *brit habat*, "covenant of the daughter," the recently introduced rite for infant girls, is a joyous welcoming and naming ceremony, an infant son's *brit milah* is "elemental, mysterious, incomprehensible and awe-ful" (sic).

The warning implicit in the preface is repeated: Although a circumcision should mean "joy" and "celebration," parents may feel "more confusion and fear than happiness." But comfort is on the way; she will inform them about the "whys" and "hows" of the rite — to reduce their "fears" and enhance the "rejoicing."[46]

A brief discussion of biblical and rabbinic interpretations follows, but Diamant obviously doesn't expect these to offer much enlightenment or solace. The "most striking line" in the liturgy, she notes, is the passage about wallowing in blood. This she interprets as a reminder of the "physical reality" of life, including "danger, dread, and death as well as spiritual aspirations." She notes that the "earthy, disquieting words" often go untranslated at a circumcision, or may even be replaced with less disturbing biblical or talmudic quotations. As for the most pressing question — why there should be such obsession with bloodshed in a welcoming ceremony for an infant — this author has no answer.

By the time prospective parents reach the section on "Modern Questions," they might well be on edge. But little relief is in sight. "Is it safe?" asks Diamant. "Will my baby suffer?" Well, she assures readers, Jewish infants have survived the procedure for 3500 years (an exaggeration of at least one thousand years, and with no information on hazards or survival rates). And after all, she continues, a religion centered on "the sanctity of life and health" would hardly require anything injurious to an infant. Complications (unspecified) are "extremely rare," and infection is unlikely because "the site of the cut is well supplied with blood." With regard to pain and suffering Diamant has "no definitive answer." Perhaps, she says, offering the lame explanations one often hears, exposure to "cold air" and being placed on his back may cause the infant as much distress as excision of the foreskin. Be that as it may, she concludes, one must acknowledge the "discomfort" experienced by *parents* — which seems to return her to more manageable territory.

Should one entrust this unsettling business to a mohel or to a physician? While the mohel is often envisioned as "a doddering old man," physicians enjoy "enormous respect." But be forewarned: medical circumcisions are often performed by "inexperienced residents" who may be "doing a few babies one after another." Moreover, if one chooses the medical route, religious protocol still calls for a ritual procedure: *hatafat dam habrit*, "shedding blood of the covenant" (translated by Diamant as "ritual drawing of blood from the site of the circumcision"), pricking the foreskin remnant with a needle to draw a drop of blood, accompanied by recitation of appropriate liturgy.[47]

In case parents are not yet sufficiently reassured, Diamant adds commentary on "symbolic castration" and "substitute for infant sacrifice" — lines of thought, she muses, leading one to ask: "Why haven't we abandoned so barbaric a practice altogether?" Her answer: If we discontinue circumcision, "we stop being Jews" — a familiar but baseless assertion.[48] However, this author — earnest and well intentioned, but out of her depth here — may be excused for inability to provide an adequate guide for the perplexed.

The same can hardly be said for Jacob Neusner, former director of a major Judaic Studies program at Brown University, an ordained rabbi, and a distinguished authority on early rabbinic Judaism and rabbinic literature. An extraordinarily prolific author, Neusner has written, in addition to countless scholarly volumes, a number of books addressed to general audiences. In *The Enchantments of Judaism*, on Jewish "rites of transformation," he defines his main audience as Jews of every kind, observant or not, who seek better understanding of "the reality of living Judaism." (He defines himself as a centrist, "closer to the Reform than the Hasidic.")[49]

Struggling to display the "enchantment" in circumcision, Neusner sounds as uneasy and ambivalent as Anita Diamant. Although the operation is "a minor surgical rite, of dubious medical value," he begins, it is nevertheless "the mark of the renewal of the agreement between God and Israel, the covenant carved into the flesh of the penis of every Jewish male — and nothing less." As for why a covenant must be carved into an infant penis, he offers only the vague assurance that the ritual liturgy (not the genital surgery) is "the medium of enchantment" that somehow transforms the business of foreskin removal and creates a spiritual experience for the child's parents: "an event heavy with meaning: a metaphor for something more, for something that transcends." (Unlike some Orthodox commentators, he makes no such claim for the infant's experience.) Then he retreats into an anecdote about his own son's circumcision. When his wife's father, holding the child in the role of *sandek*, sat on the dining room table, it collapsed, sending baby and surgical instruments to the floor. Neusner assures readers that the child survived "nicely" and grew up to play rugby for Columbia — a point repeated, as we'll see, in his closing remarks.[50]

"Enchantment," Neusner continues, "works in a mysterious way to make us do things we should not ordinarily do, to see things we commonly do not perceive." Taking for granted that we know what "things" we would rather not do, he explains what (Jewish) witnesses are intended to "perceive" during the surgery:

> We see ourselves as — in the setting of Judaism — God sees us: a family beyond time, joined by blood of not pedigree but circumcision; a genealogy framed by fifty generations of loyalty to the covenant in blood; and a birth from the union of the womb of a Jewish woman with the circumcised penis of her husband. This is the fruit of the womb — my son, my son, my son."[51]

Aside from the confusing syntax, what are we to make of such an attempt at explanation? Why the startling reference to union of womb with circumcised penis? As the author knows very well, Orthodox Jewish doctrine holds that the child of a Jewish woman is Jewish by birth, even if the father is a genitally intact Buddhist or Hindu. Moreover, there is the central question, surely on the mind of any parent seeking instruction: Why foreskin removal? Moreover, why does a spiritual covenant, understandable only by adults, require infant bloodshed — and from the penis of all places? As for the bizarre capstone, the triple invocation to "my son," might this signify admission of his own anxiety attendant on the entire procedure? Perhaps I should repeat: Jacob Neusner is one of the most accomplished Jewish scholars of our time. This retreat into vaguely mystical commentary seems uncharacteristic.

Neusner focuses on several features of the rite. First is the passage from Numbers about Phinehas (here Phineas) and the "pact of peace." Rather than dealing with the story straightforwardly, he quotes the comments by Lifsa Schachter which I cited earlier: that Phinehas gratified the Lord by punishing "sexual licentiousness and idolatry." Neusner doesn't explain how this message might enchant parents, let alone infants.

Turning to the blessing recited by the father immediately after "the *mohel* takes the knife and cuts the foreskin," Neusner offers another interpretation in the same vein: "What I do is like what Abraham did. Things are more than what they seem....my fatherhood is like Abraham's."

Finally, "yet a further occasion of enchantment": the prayer asking that the Lord rescue the child from the pit; in Neusner's translation, "save the beloved of our flesh from destruction." The message here:

> The covenant is not a generality; it is specific, concrete, fleshly. It is, moreover, meant to accomplish a specific goal...and that is to secure a place for the child, a blessing for the child. By virtue of the rite, the child enters the covenant: he enters that unseen 'Israel' that through blood enters an agreement with God. Then the blessing of the covenant is owing to the child. For covenants or contracts cut both ways.[52]

In short, the child purchases redemption and divine blessing with his genital blood.

Neusner concludes with additional musing, returning to the scene of his son's circumcision. The blessings accompanying the rite literally enchant:

> I am no longer in the here and the now; time is other than what I thought....The action is not the cutting of the flesh but the covenant of circumcision. And present are my wife and my father-in-law and my baby son on the floor, surrounded by knives and gauze. Present here, too, is the statement that we are

Israel — yet, in the here and now, the dazed father; the bemused, enchanted grandfather; the sturdy son. Varsity rugby for Columbia indeed![53]

This seems to be the ultimate message: that Jewish parents must not be overwhelmed by feelings of discomfort — or, even worse, fears that this operation may diminish the masculinity of their sons. Nor should they be concerned that the experience leaves them feeling "dazed." They can feel confident that their sons are not permanently damaged, that they will grow up to be just as "sturdy" as they had been in their intact state.[54]

Lest it appear that Neusner may have stumbled where others stride with assurance, we turn finally to *Becoming a Jewish Parent*, by another prominent rabbi-scholar, Daniel Gordis. While admitting that circumcision can be an unpleasant experience, he informs (or misinforms) us that although the event may seem "confusing," it is "not a terribly complicated ceremony" after all. But why is it considered so necessary, and what does it really mean? In order to understand the "power" of circumcision, he continues, we must acknowledge that "the whole idea makes people very uncomfortable" — which explains why they "often make silly comments" and "why the *mohel* opens with a joke." His own anxiety is already manifest: "There's a palpable tension in the room. The baby is so small, so vulnerable, so innocent. How can we explain the tradition's stipulation that we circumcise him? Now? In this way?" "Let's admit it," he continues, although most Jewish parents circumcise their infant sons, "it would be an exaggeration to say that they want to.[55]

Next (like Neusner) he shifts to a personal memory — actually a confession. Though he had attended "hundreds" of circumcisions, when it came to circumcising his own son, he "didn't know what was coming" — that is, he wasn't prepared for the disconcerting sight of the aftermath: the infant's "red and swollen" penis. During the week before the circumcision he had been changing diapers, but at his first attempt afterward he was "too upset to finish." He left the task to his wife and waited about a week before even looking again. When a second son arrived, he was again "on diaper duty" for the first week, but after the circumcision was again "granted a reprieve," leaving his wife to endure what he could not. In brief, this candid, well-intentioned rabbi, who had attended innumerable circumcisions, finally realized why parents are so "conflicted" about submitting their newborn sons to genital surgery.

Gordis's "discomfort" led him to think more about why male Jewish infants must begin life with such a traumatic experience. Of course, God commanded it, but that won't satisfy everyone. Feeling that there must be something more, he turns to the circumcision liturgy for answers — and gets no further than the passage about Phinehas. "What a strange way to begin the *berit milah!*" he exclaims, now beginning to sound as though he might prefer another profession. Why such a "strange introduction?" Having chosen to retell the story of what readers surely perceive as a vicious double murder, Gordis, squirming almost visibly, repeats his question — as though he doesn't know any better than we do how to deal with it: "Now, why in the world would the *berit milah* start with a story like that?" Well, we have to try to "think about this creatively," he urges, try to understand it "on its own terms." But his interpretive effort is so painfully convoluted that no sensible reader could feel reassured. Maybe, he proposes, the rite acknowledges our "tension and anxiety" and encourages us to ask: "What in life is so sacred that we would risk all for it?" Do we believe so deeply in some "causes" that nothing and no one can discourage us?

Although hoping that "we'll never have to kill for something we believe in" (i.e., emulate Phinehas!), he continues, perhaps it's "not a bad idea" to ask what would lead us to do so. In particular, does anything in "the *Jewish world*" matter that much to us — and could Judaism have survived this long if some of us hadn't been willing to sacrifice everything "to keep the enterprise going?" We're asking "tough questions" here, with no easy answers; but might it be that the rite of circumcision is Judaism's way of making us think about tough questions? Or perhaps "the whole point" is to make us "feel uncomfortable" (us, not the infant!). After all, we don't go through with this because we want to; "in fact, we really *don't*." We do it because we must acknowledge that the child is not actually ours: "In some strange [that adjective again] but palpable way, he belongs to the Jewish people." Incidentally, since entering the covenant is "serious business," tell the mohel: no jokes, please. The "tension" has to be "healthy, productive." The rabbi closes by throwing up his hands: "Make the most of it."[56]

Phinehas was apparently more than enough for this embattled author, who wisely omitted consideration of the "tough questions" posed by references to wallowing in blood and rescue from destruction. That matter aside, though, what are we to make of these peculiar documents, particularly those by the two rabbis? Is this really the best they could offer? Perhaps it is significant that each turned so quickly to reminiscence and confessed so candidly to personal distress. What is most remarkable is that, having undertaken to explain Jewish ritual traditions to a largely Jewish-American audience, both were stymied when they came up against Judaism's most problematic tradition.

Not everyone, though, is so ambivalent. Parents accustomed to turning to the Internet for information have "Mazel Tov," the website of Raphael Malka, a rabbi-mohel practicing in the Washington, DC area. For Rabbi Malka, blessed with a cheerful frame of mind, celebration is the order of the day — even for the infant. Circumcision, he informs readers, is a "joyous occasion in a baby's life and that of his family," a way for parents to thank God for sending them the "tender new arrival," their "*bundle from heaven*."

No one these days "questions the desirability of circumcision," he assures us, since it is now "standard hygienic practice." But of course only a properly trained mohel can convert a "surgical act" into a religious experience.[57]

Since circumcision, he continues, "has a great spiritual effect on the child," the operator must be not only medically qualified but also "religiously authorized." Enemies of Judaism have tried many times to eliminate circumcision, and of course now there are those who want to replace the religious rite with a spiritually meaningless hospital procedure. For such potential defectors Malka has a challenge: "*Shall we, through indifference, neglect a sacred rite which our forefathers have preserved at all cost?*" If your answer is a determined no, call or fax the rabbi at the numbers provided.[58]

4. CONCLUSION

Here, then, we have the kind of information available to Jewish-American parents seeking guidance on whether they should ritually circumcise their infant sons. Let me now briefly review what we know about the diversity of Jewish Americans. First and foremost is the very fact of their diversity. Only about 6% belong to Orthodox congregations; the Reform movement, already popular, is gaining ground, mainly at the expense of the middle-of-the-road Conservatives; and there is also a growing number of those who identify as secular or non-affiliated. To be sure, there is some movement in the opposite direction, most evident in a slight increase in the ultra-Orthodox cohort and in recent efforts by the Reform rabbinate to revive elements of formal ritual observance (e.g., dietary regulations) that were abandoned generations ago. But rabbinic recommendations are only that, and average Reform congregants are unlikely to adopt inconvenient practices that have never been part of their lives. Moreover, thanks to the Cohen and Eisen study, we know now that even individuals in the middle ranges of religious and ethnic commitment are disinclined to accept the idea that ritual practices are divinely ordained and must be obeyed without question. To the contrary, they express typically American insistence on individual choice and responsibility, declaring that they feel free to decide on the appropriateness of particular kinds of ritual behavior for their personal spiritual lives.

What, then, is their attitude toward commemorating Abraham's covenant by removing infant foreskins? As we've seen, Jewish-American sociologists are largely silent on this question, which in itself says a great deal. It appears that circumcision is taken so completely for granted, lies so far beyond critical examination, that sociologists, along with almost everyone else, either seldom think to ask about the practice or view such questions as out of bounds. Wondering why this is so carries us even further a field from "hard" data; but judging from what we've now learned from the popular literature on Jewish circumcision, it seems that the subject is so laden with ambivalence and discomfort that few feel comfortable even mentioning it, let alone asking the obvious questions.

The small percentage of Jewish Americans who identify as strictly Orthodox will undoubtedly continue to practice ritual circumcision into the indefinite future. In an obvious effort to counter the popular acceptance of hospital circumcisions, both the Reform and Conservative movements have been certifying physician-mohels, and some parents are turning to these practitioners as "compromise" solutions to the circumcision dilemma. But nearly all of the minimally religious or frankly secular majority have long since opted for non-ritual hospital circumcision, simply because it is "the American thing to do." They choose circumcision for their infant sons not to "inscribe" difference on their genitals but to ensure that they look no different from their fathers and their peers, Jewish and Gentile. Asked why they favor the practice, a few may offer a vaguely ethnic answer: "It's one of the oldest Jewish customs," or "It makes the boy Jewish" (or "Doesn't it make the boy Jewish?"). Most will speak about "cleanliness" or about looking like everyone else. Hardly anyone will mention preserving a covenant — and the word "sacrifice" will never come up.

I would argue, therefore, that for all immediate purposes the campaign to end infant circumcision in America should ignore Jewish Americans, or at least avoid viewing them as a relentlessly intransigent population. We should continue to focus attention on "routine" hospital circumcision. When that misguided practice has ended, large numbers of Jewish-American parents will begin to think critically about whether to retain an archaic rite with nothing to recommend it to the rational mind.

REFERENCES

1. Glazer N. American Judaism, 2nd ed. Chicago: University of Chicago Press; 1972. pp. 54-5. Reform Jews in nineteenth-century Germany were sharply divided on whether or not to retain the practice. See Katz J. The struggle over preserving the rite of circumcision in the first part of the nineteenth century. In: Katz J. Divine Law in Human Hands: Case Studies in Halakhic Flexibility. Jerusalem: Magnes Press; 1998. pp. 320-56.
2. An extensive study conducted in 1995-96 among respondents self-identified as affiliated with a denomination yielded the following percentages; the first number refers to members of congregations, the second to non-members. Orthodox: 6, 2; Conservative: 18, 15; Reform: 16, 22; Other: 2, 19. Note that these percentage figures do not include the large numbers of non-affiliated persons. Note also that 58% of the respondents claiming

"affiliation" do not actually belong to a congregation. Cohen SM. Assessing the vitality of Conservative Judaism in North America: evidence from a survey of synagogue members. In: Wertheimer J, editor. Jews in the Center: Conservative Synagogues and Their Members. New Brunswick (NJ) and London: Rutgers University Press; 2000. pp. 13-35. [here, p. 16.]

3. "The most important aspect of recent American Jewish history has been the transformation of American Jews into Jewish Americans." Shapiro ES. A Time for Healing: American Jewry Since World War II. Baltimore and London: The Johns Hopkins University Press; 1992. p. 254.

4. For representative studies, see Wertheimer J. A People Divided: Judaism in Contemporary America. New York: Basic Books; 1993 and Heilman SC. Portrait of American Jews: The Last Half of the 20th Century. Seattle and London: University of Washington Press; 1995.

5. Cohen SM and AM Eisen. The Jew Within: Self, Family, and Community in America. Bloomington and Indianapolis: Indiana University Press; 2000.

6. Cohen SM and AM Eisen. The Jew Within: Self, Family, and Community in America. Bloomington and Indianapolis: Indiana University Press; 2000. pp. 7, 11.

7. I wrote to Arnold Eisen asking why there was no mention of circumcision. He sent a gracious reply, acknowledging that neither he nor Steven Cohen could explain their failure to include even one question, other than that they "simply forgot to do so." Letter of 19 June 2001. Assuming (as I do) that this was a frank and honest answer, it is mystifying. These highly experienced scholars asked about such matters as participation in Jewish study groups, visiting Israel, candle lighting, and Christmas trees, but asked nothing about a universally recognized Jewish practice that has been controversial for more than a century. Although professional Jewish Studies scholars have to be cautious when discussing circumcision, including one or two questions among dozens would have implied nothing about personal beliefs. Is circumcision taken so thoroughly for granted that even those studying Jewish belief and practice never think to mention it?

8. In a study published in 1991, Steven M. Cohen reported that 55% of respondents to a survey said that they thought it "extremely important" that their *grandsons* be ritually circumcised, and another 18% called it "very important"–even though only 33% considered it "extremely important" that their children marry another Jew. Cited in Neusner J. Fortress Introduction to American Judaism. Minneapolis: Fortress Press; 1994. p. 45.

9. For a detailed analysis of the myth of Abraham's covenant, see Hoffman LA. Covenant of Blood: Circumcision and Gender in Rabbinic Judaism. Chicago and London: The University of Chicago Press; 1996. chap. 2.

10. Hoffman LA. Covenant of Blood: Circumcision and Gender in Rabbinic Judaism. Chicago and London: The University of Chicago Press; 1996. p. 80. The quoted phrase is italicized in Hoffman's text.

11. In a cross-cultural study of "reproductive rituals," Karen and Jeffery Paige argue that circumcision "is a surveillance ritual by which members of a strong fraternal interest group [i.e., men united in a male-centered collective], particularly the most influential members, assess and minimize the likelihood of fission [i.e., departure from the collective unit] by requiring a public demonstration of loyalty of any man who has a son." The father demonstrates that he is "willing to trust others with his and his family's most valuable political asset, his son's penis." Paige KE and JM Paige. The Politics of Reproductive Ritual. Berkeley, Los Angeles, and London: University of California Press; 1981. pp. 122-66 [here, pp. 148-9, 147]. Note also their discussion of the "ancient Hebrews," pp. 134-9.

12. Fathers and sons, not mothers and not daughters. As Hoffman demonstrates, the entire rite is characterized by "extreme sexist symbolism;" it is by and for men alone. Hoffman LA.

Covenant of Blood: Circumcision and Gender in Rabbinic Judaism. Chicago and London: The University of Chicago Press; 1996. p. 210.

13. Hoffman LA. Covenant of Blood: Circumcision and Gender in Rabbinic Judaism. Chicago and London: The University of Chicago Press; 1996. pp. 69-73. His version of the rite is based on Birnbaum P. Daily Prayer Book: Ha-Siddur Ha-Shalem. New York: Hebrew Publishing Company; 1949. pp. 741-4, and Goldin HE. Hamadrikh: The Rabbi's Guide. Revised edition. New York: Hebrew Publishing Company; 1956. pp. 33-7, both of which I have also consulted. Krohn PJ. Bris Milah: Circumcision. Brooklyn, NY: Mesorah Publications, Ltd.; 1985. pp. 118-37. An authority on Jewish religious denominations characterizes Mesorah as "identified with right-wing Orthodoxy" and "arguably the largest publisher of Jewish books today." Wertheimer J. A People Divided: Judaism in Contemporary America. New York: Basic Books; 1993. p. 120.

14. JPS Hebrew-English Tanakh. Philadelphia: Jewish Publication Society; 1999.

15. Numbers 25: 10-12; JPS Hebrew-English Tanakh. Philadelphia: Jewish Publication Society; 1999. p. 343.

16. The *sandek*, who is expected to be a "pious" man, may be the child's grandfather, a relative, or perhaps a close family friend.

17. Translations differ in details; mine derives from Hoffman LA. Covenant of Blood: Circumcision and Gender in Rabbinic Judaism. Chicago and London: The University of Chicago Press; 1996. p. 71, and the three other sources cited in note 13. Erich Isaac, an anthropologist, has explained the connection between cutting animals or objects in half and confirming covenants or agreements. Isaac E. Circumcision as a covenant rite. Anthropos 1964;59:444-56.

18. See Hoffman LA. Covenant of Blood: Circumcision and Gender in Rabbinic Judaism. Chicago and London: The University of Chicago Press; 1996. p. 35. Jon Levenson revives this argument in a reactionary article in the "neo-conservative" periodical Commentary. Levenson JD. The new enemies of circumcision. Commentary 2000;109(3):29-36. [here, p. 35.] Levenson does not mention his own study of child sacrifice, cited in note 29 below.

19. Krohn PJ. Bris Milah: Circumcision. Brooklyn, NY: Mesorah Publications, Ltd.; 1985. pp. 118-9.

20. Numbers 25. JPS Hebrew-English Tanakh. Philadelphia: Jewish Publication Society; 1999. pp. 343-4. The story appears to say that a branch of the Midianites were residing in Moabite territory and sharing their worship of Baal-peor.

21. Krohn PJ. Bris Milah: Circumcision. Brooklyn, NY: Mesorah Publications, Ltd.; 1985. p. 118.

22. Wolfson ER. Circumcision and the divine name: a study in the transmission of esoteric doctrine. Jewish Quarterly Review 1987;78:77-112. [here, pp. 102-3.] Moses's wife was said to be the daughter of Jethro, a Midianite priest. I know of no text examining the question of whether this "intermarriage" contaminated his phallus.

23. Schachter L. Reflections on the Brit Mila ceremony. Conservative Judaism 1986; 38(4):38-41. [here, p. 40.]

24. JPS Hebrew-English Tanakh. Philadelphia: Jewish Publication Society; 1999, p. 762. The passage is repeated in I Kings 19:13-14. Schachter cites I Kings 20, but this seems to be an error.

25. Schachter L. Reflections on the Brit Mila ceremony. Conservative Judaism 1986;38(4):38-41. [here, p. 41.]; author's emphasis.

26. Hoffman LA. Covenant of Blood: Circumcision and Gender in Rabbinic Judaism. Chicago and London: The University of Chicago Press; 1996. pp. 112-21. [here, p. 121.]

27. Hoffman LA. Covenant of Blood: Circumcision and Gender in Rabbinic Judaism. Chicago and London: The University of Chicago Press; 1996. p. 120.

28. Krohn translates the phrase as "rescue the beloved...from destruction" — somewhat less accurate but to the point. The Hebrew term, *shachat*, means "pit." Krohn PJ. Bris Milah: Circumcision. Brooklyn, NY: Mesorah Publications, Ltd.; 1985. p. 127.

29. Levenson JD. The Death and Resurrection of the Beloved Son: The Transformation of Child Sacrifice in Judaism and Christianity. New Haven: Yale University Press; 1993. pp. 43-52. For the possible connection with circumcision, see especially pp. 48-52. Orthodox Jews perform a rite called "Redemption of the First-Born" (*pidyon ha-ben*) on the 31st day of a male child's life; the literal translation of *pidyon* is "ransom." They pay a man supposedly descended from the priestly caste (a *kohen*) the equivalent of five ancient shekels (now interpreted as five silver dollars), ostensibly to commemorate the "redemption" of the boy from service in the Temple. Holding the coins over the child's head, the *kohen* says, "This instead of that, this in exchange for that, this is given up for that." Birnbaum P. Daily Prayer Book: Ha-Siddur Ha-Shalem. New York: Hebrew Publishing Company; 1949. pp. 751-2. Levenson translates the key term in the third phrase, *machul*, more accurately as "commutation" (p. 47)–hence, "this is commutation for that." The biblical passage underlying the rite is as follows: "You shall give Me the first-born among your sons. You shall do the same with your cattle and your flocks; seven days it shall remain with its mother; on the eighth day you shall give it to me" (Exod. 22:28-29). Levenson observes that of all biblical passages that "have been deemed offensive, none has been deemed so more often than this one, and none has generated greater resistance to a literal interpretation" (p. 3); later he calls it "a hideous demand" (p. 17). Rabbi Daniel Gordis likens the rite to circumcision, repeating a comment to be quoted later in this paper: "it's a reminder that we know the child isn't really ours....In some powerful way, he is owned by the Jewish people." Gordis D. Becoming a Jewish Parent. New York: Three Rivers Press; 1999. p. 300. He leaves readers to wonder about the "powerful way."

30. Levenson JD. The Death and Resurrection of the Beloved Son: The Transformation of Child Sacrifice in Judaism and Christianity. New Haven: Yale University Press; 1993. p. 13. A penetrating study by Carol Delaney explains the thematic connection between Abraham's circumcision and his willingness to sacrifice Isaac. Delaney C. Abraham on Trial: The Social Legacy of Biblical Myth. Princeton, NJ: Princeton University Press; 1998.

31. Levenson JD. The Death and Resurrection of the Beloved Son: The Transformation of Child Sacrifice in Judaism and Christianity. New Haven: Yale University Press; 1993. chap. 2. Day J. Molech: A God of Human Sacrifice from the Old Testament. Cambridge: Cambridge University Press; 1989. Generally accepted biblical references include Lev.18:21, Lev. 20:2-5, Jer. 7:31, Jer. 19:5, Jer. 32:35, II Kings 23:10.

32. Day J. Molech: A God of Human Sacrifice from the Old Testament. Cambridge: Cambridge University Press; 1989, chap. 2 and pp. 83-4. He suggests that the name Hinnom is related to *Gehenna*, a term close in meaning to *She'ol*.

33. Levenson JD. The Death and Resurrection of the Beloved Son: The Transformation of Child Sacrifice in Judaism and Christianity. New Haven: Yale University Press; 1993. p. 18. That conclusion is seconded by Susan Niditch: "While there is still considerable controversy about the matter...the consensus of scholars over the last decade concludes that child sacrifice was a part of ancient Israelite religion, to large segments of Israelite communities of various periods." Niditch S. War in the Hebrew Bible. New York and Oxford: Oxford University Press; 1993. p. 47.

34. Jer. 7:30-31, 19:5. JPS Hebrew-English Tanakh. Philadelphia: Jewish Publication Society; 1999. pp. 1026, 1057.

35. Levenson JD. The Death and Resurrection of the Beloved Son: The Transformation of Child Sacrifice in Judaism and Christianity. New Haven: Yale University Press; 1993. pp. 50-2.
36. Ezekiel 16:3-9, 14. JPS Hebrew-English Tanakh. Philadelphia: Jewish Publication Society; 1999. p. 1181.
37. Friedlander G, editor and translator. *Pirkei de Rabbi Eliezer.* New York: Benjamin Blom; 1971. p. 204.
38. Friedlander G, editor and translator. *Pirkei de Rabbi Eliezer.* New York: Benjamin Blom; 1971. p. 210. Parentheses in original.
39. Hoffman LA. Covenant of Blood: Circumcision and Gender in Rabbinic Judaism. Chicago and London: The University of Chicago Press; 1996. pp. 38-9, 109.
40. Hoffman LA. Covenant of Blood: Circumcision and Gender in Rabbinic Judaism. Chicago and London: The University of Chicago Press; 1996. p. 91; his emphasis. Hoffman suggests that Jews may be reluctant to recognize the association of wine with blood for two reasons: Christian symbolism associated with the "Last Supper" and medieval accusations that Jews required the blood of Christian boys for Passover matzah (pp. 90-1).
41. Eilberg-Schwartz H. The Savage in Judaism: An Anthropology of Israelite Religion and Ancient Judaism. Bloomington (IN): Indiana University Press; 1990. chap. 6.
42. In a book to be discussed briefly in note 53 below, Jacob Neusner comments that few Jewish Americans understand the circumcision liturgy or care about having it performed with strict correctness; most prefer "to do it [i.e., go through with the child's circumcision] with their eyes closed." Neusner J. Fortress Introduction to American Judaism. Minneapolis: Fortress Press; 1994. pp. 78-86. [here, p. 79.]
43. Yet another question comes to mind: Why must the infant be circumcised on the eighth day after birth? (This means one week later, since the day of birth is counted as first of the eight.) The answer, in brief, is that in the rabbinic system of thought, male blood is sacred and pure, while female blood, as shed during menstruation and childbirth, is the ultimate pollution. Hence, the child must wait for a week until it has been cleansed of maternal blood. In Leviticus 12:2-5, a verse mandating circumcision on the eighth day is inserted into a text on cleansing of women and "blood purification" after childbirth. Archer LJ. Bound by blood: circumcision and menstrual taboo in post-exilic Judaism. In: Soskice JM, editor. After Eve. London: Collins Marshall Pickering; 1990. pp. 38-61. Another possible interpretation would focus on the command that first-born sons be redeemed on the eighth day, as discussed above, note 29.
44. For more on the *Berit Mila* Board, see Glick LB. Jewish circumcision: an enigma in historical perspective. In: Denniston GC, Hodges FM, and Milos MF, editors. Understanding Circumcision: A Multi-Disciplinary Approach to a Multi-Dimensional Problem. New York: Kluwer Academic/Plenum Publishers; 2001. pp. 19-54. [here, pp. 45-7.]
45. Diamant A. The Jewish Baby Book. New York: Summit Books; 1988. pp. 18-9.
46. Diamant A. The Jewish Baby Book. New York: Summit Books; 1988. pp. 105, 107-8.
47. Diamant A. The Jewish Baby Book. New York: Summit Books; 1988. pp. 111-3.
48. Diamant A. The Jewish Baby Book. New York: Summit Books; 1988. pp. 115-6. Diamant offers several versions of the liturgy. Her standard version (pp. 124-7) includes the passages on rescue from the pit (sanitized to "protect this child from all misfortune") and on wallowing in blood ("Because of your blood you shall live!"). She also offers two "new liturgies" (pp. 133-41). The second speaks entirely in comfortable platitudes: love, compassion, harmony, and so on, ignoring the question of how these might be nurtured by removal of infant foreskins.

49. Neusner J. The Enchantments of Judaism: Rites of Transformation from Birth through Death. New York: Basic Books; 1987. pp. 5-6.
50. Neusner J. The Enchantments of Judaism: Rites of Transformation from Birth through Death. New York: Basic Books; 1987. pp. 43-5.
51. Neusner J. The Enchantments of Judaism: Rites of Transformation from Birth through Death. New York: Basic Books; 1987. p. 46.
52. Neusner J. The Enchantments of Judaism: Rites of Transformation from Birth through Death. New York: Basic Books; 1987. pp. 50-1. Although the word "cut" sounds like an unfortunate choice here, it recalls the biblical term "to cut a covenant," mentioned in note 17 above.
53. Neusner J. The Enchantments of Judaism: Rites of Transformation from Birth through Death. New York: Basic Books; 1987. p. 52; "the here and the now" sic. In an introductory book published a few years later by a Christian press and addressed mainly to non-Jewish readers, Neusner explained that the "enchantments" book answered the question of how Jewish rituals "work" to achieve "transformation." The section on circumcision (pp. 78-86) repeats some material from the earlier book and seems equally disturbing. Performing this "blood rite" in a "religious setting," Neusner says, "makes people (particularly males) confront the stark, naked reality of the faith – blood and flesh and all." He acknowledges, however, that many Jewish Americans "find implausible the message of the liturgy" and simply want to get the business done with minimal personal involvement. He concludes on a mystifying note: Since the European Jewish past came to an end with the Holocaust, for Jewish Americans "there is no past, except in rite. So why should blood repel, when blood is all there is, and when, after all, it all ended in blood....The blood of the covenant is right and true: the covenant really was, and remains, a covenant of blood, in all senses and aspects." Neusner J. Fortress Introduction to American Judaism. Minneapolis: Fortress Press; 1994. [here, pp. viii-ix, 78, 86.]
54. Note that the parents in Diamant's book are also "dazed." Sander L. Gilman has pointed out that Europeans viewed Jewish men as "uncanny, in that they superficially appear to be males but are not because of the altered form of the genitalia." Jewish men were thought to be weakened and emasculated. Gilman quotes Freud: "Circumcision is unconsciously equated with castration." Gilman SL. Freud, Race, and Gender. Princeton (NJ): Princeton University Press; 1993. Chapter 2: The construction of the male Jew. [here, pp. 49, 83.]
55. Gordis D. Becoming a Jewish Parent. New York: Three Rivers Press, 1999; pp. 295-6. I think Gordis defines his affiliation as Conservative, but I'm not certain.
56. Gordis D. Becoming a Jewish Parent. New York: Three Rivers Press, 1999; pp. 297-9; his emphasis and his spelling of *brit*.
57. Malka R. Rabbi Malka's Brit Milah Page–Mazel Tov. http://look.net/ForYou/malka/. p. 1; his emphasis. The text has "hygeinic."
58. Malka R. Rabbi Malka's Brit Milah Page–Mazel Tov. http://look.net/ForYou/malka/. pp. 2-4; his emphasis.

Chapter 13

THE GROWING JEWISH CIRCUMCISION DEBATE
A Psychosocial Critique

Ronald Goldman, Ph.D.
Executive Director, Circumcision Resource Center. Boston, MA,

Abstract: In recent years, circumcision has developed into a controversial, emotional issue among some American Jews, with articles in Jewish periodicals revealing deep disagreement about the practice. After reviewing a few of the contemporary reasons for the increasing doubts some Jews have about circumcision, and the responses of circumcision advocates, psychosocial theory is applied to explain the widely different views. The functions and characteristics of belief systems support this discussion. Other topics include motivations and meanings underlying circumcision advocates' mistaken suspicions of anti-Semitism among leading circumcision critics, the role of women in questioning circumcision, and the long-term international significance of shifting circumcision sentiments in the Jewish community.

Key words: Circumcision, psychology, psychosocial theory, Judaism, Jews, anti-Semitism

1. INTRODUCTION

In recent years, circumcision has developed into a controversial, emotional issue among some Jews. Debate about circumcision has grown partly due to information and discussion on the Internet. A popular moderated online newsgroup for Jewish parents has detailed instructions about what messages regarding circumcision are acceptable: "Because of the particularly inflammatory nature of this topic, postings about circumcision will be carefully reviewed on a case-by-case basis."[1] In addition, the Jewish press has published numerous articles about circumcision that reveal deep disagreement about the practice.[2-4]

Attitudes are associated with behaviors.[5] Circumcision in the Jewish community today is widespread. However, circumcision is not universal among Jews either inside or outside the United States. The Circumcision Resource Center, a nonprofit educational organization, has been contacted by hundreds of Jews who have not circumcised a son. Even in Israel some Jews do not circumcise, and there is an Israeli organization that publicly opposes circumcision.[6]

For many Jews, this shift has come as a surprise. New information about circumcision often conflicts with previous teachings and long-held beliefs. If our world makes sense, then there must be a coherent explanation for all the apparently contradictory information. The conflicting beliefs and opinions surrounding circumcision, together with the tenacity with which advocates and critics of circumcision hold on to their viewpoints, suggest that deep psychosocial factors are involved.

A few of the contemporary reasons for the increasing doubts some Jews have about the practice are discussed in earlier work.[7] Familiarity with these issues is necessary to understanding the context of this chapter, which reviews the responses of circumcision advocates to critics and applies psychosocial theory to explain the widely different views on the issue. Circumcision is a very complex topic, and this discussion is necessarily condensed. For more detailed information, please consult the references.

2.   PERSPECTIVE OF THIS WORK

The religious meaning of Jewish circumcision is written in the Torah where God commanded that Abraham and all Jewish males shall be circumcised as a sign of the covenant between God and the Jewish people (Genesis 17:10). For traditional Jews, this Torah commandment is the reason to circumcise. However, most Jews are unaware of the religious meaning of circumcision. Rabbi Eugene Cohen estimates that eighty percent of American Jewish circumcisions do not meet religious ritual standards.[8] According to the Council of Jewish Federations 1990 National (American) Jewish Population Survey, a majority of Jews do not consider religion to be the primary factor determining Jewish identity. Cultural and ethnic factors are rated higher. "Further analysis shows that less than five percent of all respondents consider being Jewish solely in terms of being a member of a religious group, whereas ninety percent define being Jewish as being a member of a cultural or ethnic group."[9] Only thirteen percent believe "the Torah is the actual word of God."[10] Therefore, this work is intended for those who modify Jewish practice in a way that is meaningful to them.

Non-traditional Jews generally evaluate an idea by its agreement with reason and experience. Reform Jews comprise a large proportion of this group. Eugene Borowitz, noted theologian and scholar, states that Reform Jews "believe that we serve God best by being true to our minds and consciences even where, in significant matters, they clash with our heritage."[11] Based on the above survey, a high proportion of American Jews has this perspective.

3.   CIRCUMCISION ADVOCATES REPLY

In response to literature that documents extreme pain and trauma, infant behavioral changes resulting from circumcision, risk of complications, adverse sexual effects, emotional distress of circumcised men, and anxieties and regrets of parents, Jewish circumcision advocates express their views in the American Jewish press.[12] Here are some examples.

3.1   Jewish Spectator

In an article published in *Jewish Spectator,* I explain several arguments that raise doubts about the advisability of circumcision for some Jews.[13] In a subsequent issue there are three letters in response of considerable length that support circumcision.

Rivy Kletenick, an administrator in Jewish education, focuses on the meaning of the circumcision ritual.[14] She defends circumcision by saying it is "a pure expression of devotion to God." She emphasizes "the transcendent dimension" of brit milah and the "holy words and intentions." In response to the pain argument, Kletenick "can't recall either of our two sons experiencing such pain. . . . Tough love often involves some pain. And most pain leads to growth." In response to studies on the adverse sexual and psychological consequences, Kletenick ends her letter by quoting her mother who believes that circumcised men are "all doing just fine."

Rabbi Donald Tam acknowledges that change is sometimes necessary, but "Jewish history and identity must inform change."[15] He notes that circumcision is supported for health reasons and expresses skepticism and ridicule regarding the evidence of sexual and psychological effects of circumcision.[16]

Rabbi Daniel Gordis also dismisses evidence of sexual and psychological effects of circumcision for some men, claiming that millions of people have no problem.[17] For Gordis, the ritual transmits "powerful moral and spiritual messages [that] far outweigh its minuscule medical risks."[18] He elaborates on the religious meanings for adults based on liturgy. With reference to the

Torah, he "celebrates" the anxiety of the bris as symbolic of risking for devotion to a cause.

Gordis believes that the questioning of ritual "is largely because the powerful dramas underlying them go unexplained. The solution is not to do away with the rituals, but to educate our children and ourselves better."[19] Proponents of circumcision, he states, "must begin with a reverence for tradition and be reasonably versed in the subtleties of text."[20]

These writers express little or no acknowledgment of circumcision as a cultural practice for most Jews, the infant's feelings, and ethical concerns associated with inflicting pain.

3.2   Midstream

Lisa Braver Moss, a mother of two circumcised sons, is the author of an article called "Circumcision: A Jewish Inquiry."[21] Citing medical research, Jewish principles, and personal experience, she calls attention to five points: the infant's pain, the lack of religious motivation of many Jews in choosing circumcision for their son, the infant's lack of choice, risk of complications, and the acceptability of circumcising infants as compared to older children. As a cultural Jew, Moss expresses sensitivity to those Jews who circumcise for nonreligious reasons. (She circumcised her sons so that they would look like other Jewish males, and she would avoid conflict with her husband and other Jews.) Contrary to the concerns of some circumcision advocates, she reports that questioning circumcision has strengthened her Jewish identity.

The rebuttal to this article is written by the magazine's editorial assistant, Esther Raul-Friedman.[22] She faults Moss for not adequately considering the religious or spiritual significance of brit milah. Regarding the child's lack of choice, Raul-Friedman cites Jewish law that makes it the father's responsibility. She quotes a circumciser who says that circumcision is "absolutely painless"[23] and "infants do not feel any pain"[24] and blames the pain of circumcision on the clamps used by doctors. Raul-Friedman lauds claims of medical "benefits," and asserts that circumcision "activates an inner commitment to God and His commandments."[25] Not circumcising would "deprive their son of his legacy."[26] According to one circumciser, it is a "spiritual life insurance policy." Raul-Friedman concludes "circumcision is the very foundation for the continued spiritual survival of the Jewish people."

This rebuttal refers to about two dozen Jewish text sources to explain the importance of brit milah. As with Gordis and Kletenick, these sources, and the beliefs associated with them, are not relevant to cultural Jews like Ms. Moss who circumcise for nonreligious reasons.

Those who are open to all aspects of the ritual know that spirituality is a valuable component of Judaism, but it does not require neglecting reason and experience. Rabbi Milton Steinberg explains that:

> [Judaism] places understanding among its supreme purposes, and in the further sense that it believes in knowledge as a key to understanding. But neither knowledge nor understanding is attainable without inquiry, debate, and the right to make up one's own mind. By its nature, then, Judaism is averse to formal creeds which of necessity limit and restrain thought.[27]

3.3   Commentary

Jon Levenson, a professor of Jewish studies at Harvard, responds to critics in an article titled, "The New Enemies of Circumcision."[28] This extended article calls for an extended response. With such a confrontational title, Levenson apparently feels threatened and is preparing for verbal warfare in defense of circumcision, using terms like "battle" and "struggle."

Levenson's purpose is to warn his Jewish readers of the growing threat to circumcision and the values he associates with the practice. However, most American Jews do not share his values, which come from his interpretations of Jewish texts and traditional rabbinic theology. As stated earlier, the majority of Jews associate Jewish identity with cultural and ethnic factors, do not believe the Torah is the word of God, and circumcise for nonreligious reasons.

In any case, Levenson proceeds to comment on three recent books that are critical of the practice: *Circumcision: A History of the World's Most Controversial Surgery* by David Gollaher, *Questioning Circumcision: A Jewish Perspective* by Ronald Goldman, and *Covenant of Blood* by Lawrence Hoffman. He finds little merit in any book and much to critique, disparage, and even ridicule.

Levenson distrusts Gollaher's motives and intentions, concluding that Gollaher is not a "dispassionate observer" and displays "partisanship." If Levenson wants to allege partisanship, then why not do it in a non-partisan way, and question the partisanship of rabbinic texts? In addition, would he be insisting on a "dispassionate observer" if the topic were the equivalent genital cutting of females? Obviously, anyone who cares enough to write about the advisability of circumcision has an opinion about it.

Levenson calls for "double-blind studies" to prove the harm of circumcision, but apparently accepts without question that circumcision is harmless when no such studies of long-term effects have reached that conclusion. Who has the burden of proof? Rabbi Joel Roth, professor of Talmud and rabbinics at the Jewish Theological Seminary of America, wrote, "Once the command of the covenant is no longer determinative . . . the burden of proof is not on those who ignore the ritual but on those who observe it."[29]

Regarding the severe pain of circumcision, Levenson trivializes it by supposing that the potential prevention of disease justifies the pain. Here he ignores the overwhelming worldwide opinion of national medical organizations, none of which recommend circumcision.[30-32] Instead he cites medical claims that have been either refuted or judged to be insignificant by the American Academy of Pediatrics.[33]

Questioning Circumcision: A Jewish Perspective includes detailed discussion of numerous medical, psychological, sexual, emotional, and ethical issues. With no comment on these perspectives, apparently Levenson has no specific disagreement. Instead he creates generalized straw men. For example, his inflated characterization of the book's description of circumcision as "a positively demonic force that has caused all manner of devastation"[34] provides him with a convenient target.

Levenson then selects and distorts the discussion on the potential social effects of circumcision, perhaps the most complex section of the book. This discussion is necessarily speculative because, as stated in the book, "more reports and studies would be helpful, but they are not yet available."[35] Levenson rearranges quoted phrases out of context, and then presents his reformulated statements as the book's conclusion, not speculation.[36] After attacking this straw man, Levenson apparently believes he has successfully refuted the entire book and moves on to critique *Covenant of Blood*.

According to Hoffman's reading of the classical Jewish texts, the blood of circumcision symbolized salvation. By contrast, the ancient rabbis considered women's menstrual blood to be "unclean." These opposing rabbinic attitudes toward blood were consistent with similarly conflicting attitudes toward men and women. Specifically, Hoffman finds that the early rabbis distrusted women. They wrote that women are impulsive and uncontrolled, while men have self-control. These beliefs helped to justify the continuing patriarchal control of Jewish religion and culture. Hoffman determines that circumcision has held a central place in the formation, shaping, and perpetuation of significant aspects of Jewish culture that conflicted with his feminist, egalitarian views. In reviewing Hoffman's work, Levenson comes to different conclusions based on his own interpretations of the texts, and judges Hoffman as "playing fast and loose with the data."[37]

Levenson then expresses concern about the potential social influence of the circumcision debate. He fears that nontraditional Jews will increasingly question circumcision if the general culture finds circumcision to be harmful. Apparently, he fears social pressure not to circumcise but welcomes (or ignores) social pressure to circumcise. He also notes that more than a few rabbis already question circumcision (a fact that probably gives that position more credibility with Jews) and may be unlikely to advise ambivalent Jews to follow the commandment to circumcise.

In my view, Levenson's fear is associated with his rigid position on the issue. He projects a future possibility (general culture finds circumcision to be harmful) onto the screen of his present beliefs (circumcision is good), a counter-productive exercise. It is important to understand that this is an early phase of an extended national debate. In the end, the issue will be decided carefully and deliberately based on the facts because the outcome will need public support. If the facts show that circumcision is harmless, then Levenson and other circumcision advocates have nothing to fear.

However, if the facts show, as most of the world and a significant American minority now believe, that circumcision is harmful, then those who make the circumcision decision, Jews and non-Jews alike, may not choose to inflict this harm on their sons in light of the new information available. Clearly, the arguments opposing circumcision must be compelling to persuade people to change an embedded cultural practice. If the arguments are compelling, the beliefs of reasonable people would eventually conform to the facts, and choosing not to inflict harm would be a positive development. It may be that Levenson and other circumcision advocates do not trust this process because they want assurance of a particular result, regardless of the facts.

Despite his strong advocacy, Levenson asserts only two reasons for circumcision: it is a divine commandment, and it has potential medical "benefits." Both of these reasons are open to question for many Jews. In observing the growing opposition to circumcision, Levenson is obliged to acknowledge some of the many reasons others use to question circumcision: dubious origin, conflicting medical claims, severe pain, a history of Jewish questioning of circumcision, sexist implications, human rights considerations, mutilation, doubtful rabbis, the child's perfection at birth, and the lack of the child's consent. Levenson does not consider the possibility that any issues raised by circumcision critics have merit. Others are more receptive. Most of the letters published in response to his article are critical of his views and question circumcision.[38]

4. APPLYING PSYCHOSOCIAL THEORY

Sometimes understanding communication can be enhanced by paying attention to the process in addition to the content. Therefore, the following discussion applies psychosocial theory as a tool in examining the communication process that results in the widely different views held by circumcision critics and advocates. The first theory is a widely accepted one about how people respond to inconsistencies.

4.1   Cognitive Dissonance Theory

Cognitive dissonance occurs when new information or experience is inconsistent with existing cognitions.[39-40] Recent research supports the theory of cognitive dissonance.[41-42] Cognitions may include beliefs, values, and attitudes about the environment, oneself, or one's behavior. Dissonance can result from a logical inconsistency between cognitions, inconsistencies involving cultural beliefs and practices, one specific opinion as part of a more general opinion, and past experience. Factors that affect the strength of the dissonance are as follows: the degree of discrepancy among beliefs, the number of dissonant beliefs, the number of consonant beliefs, and the importance attached to each belief.

People want coherence and consistency in their cognitions and experience. If inconsistency occurs we will try to reduce the dissonance. There are three ways to reduce dissonant beliefs: (1) reduce the importance of the dissonant beliefs (or increase the importance of the consonant beliefs), (2) add more consonant beliefs that outweigh the dissonant beliefs, or (3) change the dissonant beliefs so that they are no longer inconsistent.

When there is an inconsistency between cognitions and behavior, usually the cognitions will change. When cognitions are very resistant to change, dissonance can also be reconciled by denying or altering our experience. That is, we may perceive and accept only information that fits our cognitions.

This theory can be applied to questioning Jewish circumcision. First, dissonance is affected by the importance attached to beliefs. The circumcision advocates discussed here appear to have traditional religious beliefs. Religious beliefs have very high importance for many people. In addition, questioning circumcision for a traditional Jew is not just a matter of questioning a belief. Traditional Jews also believe that God commanded Jews to circumcise. Beliefs about God and one's relationship to God are core beliefs of the religious belief system. The religious belief system helps us define the meaning of our experience and influences how we approach life's basic problems and anxieties.[43] It provides freedom from existential concerns.[44] It is connected with our emotional needs, reflects an individual's character, needs, defenses, and conscience and is highly resistant to change.[45] Perhaps it is not surprising that those with traditional religious beliefs would be most motivated to respond to writing that questions circumcision. For them, questioning circumcision is tantamount to questioning the wisdom and authority of God and their religious belief system.

According to cognitive dissonance theory, the degree of discrepancy among beliefs affects dissonance. The discrepancy between the belief that God commanded circumcision (implying that circumcision is not harmful) and the belief that circumcision is harmful is very high. As stated by Esther Raul-Friedman, it is "unacceptable to dismiss the mitzvah of brit milah by claiming that Hashem [God] has made a mistake."[46] The tendency to avoid new information increases when the discrepancy between beliefs and experience increases.[47] Because traditional Jewish beliefs about God and circumcision are based on Jewish texts and very resistant to change, and the discrepancy with new information is high, traditional Jews have little choice but to deny or alter their experience and reject information (without appropriate consideration of the merits) that does not fit their beliefs.

Kletenick's, Gordis', and Raul-Friedman's responses provide examples of reducing cognitive dissonance by reducing the importance of (or dismissing) dissonant beliefs (empirical evidence) and increasing the importance of consonant beliefs (spiritual benefits). Levenson does the same thing by trivializing pain as compared to health claims. Kletenick also changes a dissonant belief so that it is no longer dissonant (rationalizing that pain has benefits). Gordis uses a similar approach to interpreting the anxiety of the bris (symbolic of risking for a cause rather than attending to the risk to the child). (Others, repeating arguments in Jewish texts, change a dissonant belief so that it is no longer dissonant by claiming that the sexual loss is a benefit.[48])

What about nonreligious circumcision beliefs? The attitude that circumcision is good or harmless (I am not harmed, my son is not harmed, etc.) is an important cognition for many people. Information and experience that challenge this cognition have a high discrepancy and may be avoided or denied no matter how valid and reliable they are. (See "Denial" later.) Cognitive dissonance theory says that adding consonant beliefs can reduce dissonance. The mind seeks reasons (consonant beliefs) to justify behavior. In the United States, consonant health beliefs are adopted to reduce cognitive dissonance associated with circumcision. These claims are often used by Americans and Jews, and in this review by Tam, Raul-Friedman, and Levenson. This is nothing new. Circumcision has a long American history of being promoted by medical doctors to prevent or cure dozens of ailments such as indigestion, paralysis, hernia, inflammation of the bladder, general nervousness, constipation, masturbation, penile cancer, feeblemindedness, uncleanliness, and most recently, HIV infection.[49] Consonant health beliefs change as cultural values and research results change, but the quest to reduce dissonance remains constant. Needless to say, the unending search for a problem that calls for circumcision "treatment" arouses suspicion that there are psychosocial factors at work.

Beliefs that circumcision is important because of Jewish survival, identity, and tradition may be other examples of cognitions that are used to reconcile cognitive dissonance associated with nonreligious (cultural) Jewish circumcision. Of course, since the theory says that adding more consonant beliefs reduces dissonance, traditional Jews may also choose to supplement religious belief with these beliefs.

How does this theory apply to the cognitions of circumcision critics? Based on reason and experience, dissonant (pro-circumcision) beliefs that can be argued rationally have been addressed in previous work where survival, identity, tradition, and health beliefs used to justify circumcision are shown to be either debatable at best or irrational.[50] (Using reason, circumcision critics would argue that a debatable belief is not sufficient justification to cut off someone else's body part.) Consonant beliefs about circumcision harm have documented support from authorities in relevant fields.

A key factor is that the documentation of harm is consistent with personal experience. How is the personal experience of critics (e.g., horrified at hearing the infant's cry) more valid than conflicting personal experience? Some Jews report attending a bris and not hearing the infant cry. The relationship between infant pain and vocal response needs explanation. The cry may be reduced by the affect of anesthetics given to the mother during labor.[51] These anesthetics enter the infant's body and, according to pediatrician T. Berry Brazelton, they can take over a week to leave.[52] Other factors can also account for minimal vocal response. Justin Call, infant psychologist and professor-in-chief of child and adolescent psychology at the University of California, reports that "sometimes babies who are being circumcised . . . lapse into a semi-coma."[53] Tonya Brooks, president of the International Association for Childbirth at Home and a midwife, observes, "In four of the nine circumcisions that I have seen, the baby didn't cry. He just seemed to be suddenly in a state of shock!"[54] Studies demonstrate that even though an infant may not cry during circumcision, the stress hormone level in the blood still increases dramatically, and medical researchers consider this change to be the most reliable indicator of pain response.[55] Therefore, lack of crying does not mean that the infant feels no pain. It means that he is withdrawing from unbearable pain. In addition, parents are unlikely to express any adverse response to the circumcision because these feelings are so painful and are not generally supported by the community.[56-57]

This work attempts to explain the conflict between experiences of advocates and critics with psychological theory and evidence regarding the infant's vocal response (See also "Denial" later). Circumcision advocates have not yet offered an explanation for this conflict, which would involve explaining why some people are horrified at witnessing circumcision and why they should distrust their feelings. The beliefs, values, attitudes, and experiences of circumcision critics are consistent. The dissonance for critics is not only reduced, but eliminated, not by changing cognitions but by changing the behavior, i.e., not circumcising. Based on their experience and new information, they consider this change important.

4.2   Belief Systems

Clearly, one of the sources of conflict between circumcision advocates discussed here and circumcision critics is the difference in their belief systems. Milton Rokeach, professor of psychiatry at Michigan State University, wrote a classic work on how people organize systems of belief and respond to ideas, authorities, and people.[58] He summarized that belief systems serve two conflicting needs: as a framework to understand reality and a defense against threatening aspects of reality. For open systems, the need to understand predominates, and information can be received and assessed. In closed systems, the need to protect against threats becomes stronger and the need to know becomes weaker. However, the closed mind is experienced subjectively no differently than the open mind, and preserves the illusion of the need to know.

Here are some of Rokeach's characteristics of a closed belief system:

•perception that the environment is threatening

•belief that authority is absolute

•difficulty receiving, evaluating, and acting on relevant information on its own merits

•dependency on own group's authorities

•independence of the power of authority from cognitive correctness

•large discrepancy between what is known about the belief system and what is known about those areas that lie outside the belief system (disbelief system)

•acceptance or rejection of a variety of information in total without differentiation

In applying these characteristics to the writing of circumcision advocates presented here, recall that Levenson refers to circumcision critics as "enemies," suggesting that he perceives the environment as threatening, although, among Jews, he is a member of the overwhelming majority on this issue. He and Raul-Friedman view religious authority (Jewish texts) as absolute. Raul-Friedman in particular is dependent on Jewish text authorities when the authorities on circumcision harm are found in the relevant professional literature. The conflict between text authorities and empirical studies/experience does not introduce any doubt for circumcision advocates about text authorities' power. Apparently, these writers do not know much about circumcision harm (disbelief system). Various aspects of circumcision harm are categorically rejected or ignored. It appears that advocates' difficulty in receiving and evaluating relevant information on its merits is at least partly due to a closed belief system.

4.3   Denial

The rejection of information about circumcision harm is only part of the difficulty in communication about circumcision. It is also possible to reject other pertinent experience. Freud wrote, "The tendency to forget the disagreeable seems to me to be quite general."[59] The subject of circumcision is so "disagreeable" that many people will avoid it consciously and unconsciously. In psychoanalytic theory, defense mechanisms are unconscious ways of dealing with the "disagreeable," internal emotional pain and external experience that stimulates emotional pain. Denial is a defense mechanism that involves a refusal to acknowledge certain aspects of experience. The ability of people to deny their experience is not appreciated because it is the evidence itself that is denied or interpreted to mean something else.

Denial can be amazingly effective. Pediatrician Paul Fleiss did circumcisions for ten years and says, "I never heard the baby cry."[60] Dr. Gregory Skipper, a prospective father, recognized his denial after observing a circumcision.

> I watched a circumcision being performed and immediately, without any question, knew that there was no way that I could have my newborn son tortured in such a manner. It seemed like the first time that I had ever really watched the procedure, even though I had done several dozen in medical school. The baby was absolutely panicked and exhibited the most shrill and desperate behavior one could imagine! The pediatrician performing the procedure continued his mutilation as if nothing were happening. I almost vomited.[61]

Denial may explain why Jewish ritual circumcisers can report that circumcision is "painless." The use of defense mechanisms by these circumcisers, physicians, and parents may serve, in part, to protect their self-esteem. Recognizing that they are harming an infant might cause them not to feel good about themselves. Because protecting self-esteem sometimes takes priority over being accurate or correct, potentially threatening information may be reinterpreted or dismissed.[62-63] Another example of reinterpreting an experience is that some parents may choose circumcision and deny that they have made a choice.[64] This can happen without awareness.

Those who attend a bris sometimes report that the baby did not cry. This report may be due to at least two possibilities: the baby did not cry (explained earlier) or the observer did not hear the cry. Those who witness circumcisions may deny this part of their experience. Indications of this denial can be detected empirically in the form of reduced physiological response.[65] In extreme cases a person may shut down physically by fainting. This has been observed at ritual circumcisions and hospital circumcisions.[66-68]

5.   BEYOND ANTI-SEMITISM

By denying or ignoring any merit in questions and arguments critical of circumcision, Jewish circumcision advocates are left with suspecting a hidden motivation for those who would question circumcision.[69] They need to make sense of what they perceive. How could Jews and others question a divine commandment? Levenson believes that the views of circumcision critics are affected by "Jewish self-hate" and "anti-Semitism."[70]

The indiscriminate use of these terms by more than a few Jewish leaders calls for examination and response. Jewish self-hate is a generalized feeling. If a Jew feels self-hate (A), then he is likely to dislike specific Jewish things (B). However, questioning a specific Jewish thing does not necessarily equate with generalized Jewish self-hate. As we learned in high school logic, *if A then B* does not equal *if B then A*. To further illustrate in a parallel example, some Catholics disagree with certain Catholic ideas and rituals, but they are not accused of being "self-hating Catholics." Furthermore, hate is a very strong and easily identifiable feeling. The published writing of leading Jewish critics of circumcision are generally either scholarly, factual analyses or compassionate statements that reveal intellectual, emotional, and ethical conflicts with the practice. Typically, they include expressions of appreciation for Judaism and a desire to contribute to the community, hardly the feelings of self-hating Jews.[71-74]

If one is anti-Semitic, then by definition one is hostile to Jews. The content of the writing of circumcision critics conflicts with this characterization. Published critiques of circumcision are uniformly rational investigations and/or personal explorations of a challenging subject.[75-77] If someone is anti-Semitic (A), then he is likely to dislike specific Jewish things (B). However, assuming that a critic of circumcision is anti-Semitic makes an over-generalized assumption. Again, elementary logic tells us that this reverse relationship does not follow. (Historically, some anti-Semites have been anti-circumcision, but that association does not mean that all circumcision critics are anti-Semitic.) A specific does not prove a generality. If you don't like asparagus (specific), this does not prove that you dislike all vegetables (generality). Some circumcision advocates fail to differentiate between reasonable criticism of a specific practice and a more general unjustified hostile attitude. It is possible to question the actions of a person or group without being categorically opposed to the person or group. Are those who question an American government policy anti-American? In fact, questioning an action that one believes can cause harm is more likely to be motivated by good will rather than ill will. If circumcision is harmful, then acting on awareness and knowledge of this harm is appropriate.

Simply the belief of some Jews or even the majority of Jews, that circumcision critics are anti-Semitic does not necessarily make critics anti-Semitic. Because of the nature of the topic, it may be that a majority of Jews judge that a *position* critical of circumcision is anti-Semitic. However, it may also be that this majority shrinks to a minority when the critical position is presented in a coherent, detailed, compassionate, and rational form. As previously discussed, some Jews may be so rigid in their advocacy of circumcision that they do not consider the details of opposing arguments.

More generally, minority positions may initially be judged to be anti-group by the majority of a group. However, individuals and groups can have various psychological, social, and political reasons for opposing change, and these reasons often have nothing to do with the merits of the proposed change. If the minority position later becomes the majority position, the "anti" label is not used. It seems that the "anti" label is often applied to marginalize those who have unpopular views.

Other factors can explain accusations of Jewish self-hate and anti-Semitism. For example, circumcision advocates may use these terms to exaggerate the challenge to their views in order to encourage a stronger Jewish response, to "rally the troops" to defend circumcision. Perhaps some Jewish leaders also invoke anti-Semitism in an effort to intimidate critics and suppress further debate. Virtually nobody wants to be called anti-Semitic. People may also falsely attribute their own feelings or traits to others, an act called projection. The perceived hostility by some circumcision advocates may be a projection of their own hostility toward those who express an opposing view. Overreaction may be associated with underlying fear and hypersensitivity associated with their own circumcision.[78]

Given the symbolic, religious, and cultural meaning of circumcision to Jews and the repressed feelings associated with circumcision, it is understandable that some Jews may overreact to circumcision critics.

Raising questions about Jewish circumcision may cause feelings of extreme grief or anger in certain individuals. Circumcision critics generally empathize with and respect these feelings. Certainly, it is extremely uncomfortable for some Jews to consider what it means for circumcision to be a very serious mistake. People are more likely to focus on what others have done to them, rather than to acknowledge what they have done to themselves. In addition, because of the long history of oppression against Jews in general and the Holocaust in particular, there is understandable protectiveness and distrust felt among Jews in response to criticism. For some Jews, even the slightest perceived criticism must be defended against and reciprocated. Of course, in the case of circumcision, the criticism concerns a central Jewish practice. Therefore, although being attacked as an anti-Semite or self-hating Jew may be inappropriate, it is understandable, and circumcision critics are urged to show compassion for circumcision advocates while knowing that they may respond directly and specifically with various options.

In my view, the proper response for Jews is to support each other in airing these feelings within the Jewish community. Opportunities to meet, learn, and express thoughts and feelings about circumcision in a safe and supportive environment would be helpful. Respectful and compassionate talking and listening would assist healing. While critics can respect the pain and anger of advocates, advocates can respect that critics are compelled to raise their questions out of deep caring and compassion for Jews generally and Jewish male infants in particular. Critics see Jews inflicting extreme unrecognized pain with this practice, and judge that the perpetuation of this pain is far greater than the pain that comes with confronting the issues they raise.

Tolerance and openness are needed. The previously mentioned moderated newsgroup supports tolerance by rejecting any judgmental messages "that criticize a parent for *ANY* circumcision decision made for their son."[79] Those in leadership positions in the Jewish community have a special obligation to facilitate discussion of this issue. This is more likely to happen with community encouragement and support.

The growing Jewish circumcision debate will certainly stir repressed feelings about circumcision, and discomfort is inevitable. However, this discomfort may be interpreted as a *positive* development. It is a sign of progress to feel and express discomfort about circumcision rather than continuing to avoid new information and pretend that the procedure is harmless. In any case, as we know from other experiences, avoiding discomfort in ourselves or others often serves only to perpetuate a problem.

6.   ROLE OF WOMEN

Circumcision has traditionally been the province of men, but the wisdom, feelings, and experiences of women can be particularly important to raising awareness and contributing new insights. Circumcision, like any other issue associated with childbirth and early infancy, needs to be addressed by the most sensitive, empathetic, and responsive human beings. According to a study on adult responses to infant crying, women are more likely than men to report feeling distressed.[80] The maternal instincts and experiences of women uniquely qualify them for the important responsibility of caring for infants, and newborn infants recognize, prefer, and are more responsive to their mothers.[81-82]

After a period of dormancy, maternal instincts are awakening around the question of circumcision. (There is an organization called Mothers Against Circumcision.) Following years of reflection, one mother asked, "If a women is made to distrust her most basic instinct to protect her newborn child, what feelings can she ever trust?"[83] Another mother, in conflict with her husband about circumcision, reported she "became like a mother lion protecting her cub."[84] Mothers' feelings about circumcision tend to be more open perhaps also because they are not themselves circumcised and not subject to the personal psychological motivations of circumcised men to perpetuate the practice.[85-86] A survey of randomly selected primary care physicians showed that circumcision was more often supported by doctors who were older, male, and circumcised.[87]

Recent investigations have added new reasons for women to be concerned about circumcision. According to a recent study, circumcision can adversely affect female sexual enjoyment.[88] Furthermore, any adverse psychological consequences of circumcision on males may adversely affect male-female relationships.[89] Because of the prevalence of circumcision in the United States, some potential adverse psychological effects of circumcision (known and unknown) on males may have indirect adverse social effects on women.[90]

Most of the people that call the Circumcision Resource Center seeking information or support about circumcision issues, Jewish or not, are women. Sometimes they have a conflict with a partner who insists on circumcision for their boy. We encourage women to raise the subject of circumcision early and to be patient and compassionate with mates who have resistance to reconsidering this issue.

Some mothers recognize that circumcision is irrevocable while, despite the best of intentions, their relationship with the father is not necessarily permanent. They believe that if they allowed their son to be circumcised because of the father's insistence, and then became divorced, they might feel deep regret. Other mothers report that agreeing reluctantly to a circumcision has had a long-term effect on them and affected their relationship with their child and mate. It is the one decision they wish they could take back. A few mothers feel so strongly about their child's welfare that they would do whatever it takes to protect their child from circumcision. (This kind of conflict can best be avoided by raising the topic of circumcision, along with other issues pertaining to children, before committing to the relationship.) Those in doubt believe that the conservative choice is not to circumcise. With most Jewish circumcisions taking place in hospitals, women have an important role because they sign most hospital circumcision consent forms.[91]

7.   AMERICAN-JEWISH CIRCUMCISION CONNECTION

Jewish parents are aware that circumcision is a common American practice. The United States is the only country in the world that circumcises most of its male infants for nonreligious reasons.[92] As Jews distance themselves from traditional religious beliefs, other beliefs are needed to justify circumcision. As noted earlier, cognitive dissonance theory explains that more consonant beliefs help to minimize dissonance.[93] Therefore, Jewish circumcision advocates take comfort in health claims because such claims are associated with American circumcision, and they seem to have a rational basis.[94-95] Some Jews also believe that health factors were part of the origin of Jewish circumcision. However, Jewish circumcision was never intended as a health measure.[96] Not only nonreligious Jews find the claim of health benefits appealing. Even some traditional Jews, as discussed earlier, argue that Jewish circumcision has health benefits.[97-98]

Jewish practice also influences the American practice. For example, of all the letters to the editor in response to the American Academy of Pediatrics Circumcision Policy Statement, the most strongly pro-circumcision responses were from Jewish doctors, including two who also perform Jewish ritual circumcisions.[99-101] Of course, there are also Jewish doctors that oppose circumcision, and Thomas Wiswell, a strong circumcision advocate, is not Jewish.[102] However, some of the most outspoken advocates for circumcision tend to be Jewish. This suggests a religious or cultural bias on the part of these advocates. According to a MEDLINE search, one strong Jewish advocate has been published twenty times in the medical literature on the subject of circumcision.

Regarding the medical profession's attitude toward circumcision, a physician at a major hospital in Boston who wrote the hospital's circumcision information sheet for parents defended its pro-circumcision bias by stating that "the religious aspect of circumcision plays a significant role."[103] According to this physician, discouraging circumcision would put doctors "in a position of attacking religious belief."[104] This stance suggests that religion may be a factor that inhibits the full disclosure of medical information and medical views on circumcision.

As another example, an organization that supports breastfeeding refuses to educate its membership about circumcision even though there is clear evidence that circumcision disrupts breastfeeding.[105] In defense of their inaction, the leadership observes that for some people, circumcision is a religious issue, and the leadership wants to avoid making "some parents feel unwelcome or uncomfortable."[106]

The reluctance to criticize circumcision extends to American government authorities. In response to an inquiry, a representative of the United States Department of Health and Human Services stated that, "Any attempt by any public agency to discourage non-medical circumcision could be misinterpreted as an attack on those religious groups which practice it"[107]. Later he added that, "it is not proper for our Government to adopt a policy that is directly or indirectly critical of a religious practice."[108]

8.   SIGNS OF RELIGIOUS INFLUENCE IN OTHER COUNTRIES

It is illuminating to examine the status of circumcision in other countries. Canada has a newborn circumcision rate of seventeen percent[109] Newborn circumcision in the United Kingdom is rare, and 3.8 percent of boys born there today would be circumcised by age fifteen if the current rate continues.[110] These figures suggest that the public pressure to perpetuate circumcision in these countries is minimal. Furthermore, those who create such policies in these countries, if they are male, would be more likely to have a foreskin and appreciate its value than their presumably circumcised American male counterparts. However, most of these countries' medical societies have issued somewhat more critical but tolerant statements about circumcision. With growing evidence of harm, why didn't they publish stronger statements opposing circumcision?

The Canadian situation is instructive. Activists opposed to circumcision applied for public funding to launch a court challenge aimed at banning the circumcision of baby boys. This was a national media story.[111] The group explains on its website why it proposed its challenge:

> Over the past few years many Canadian agencies, both governmental and non-governmental, have been approached by citizens on the subject of non-therapeutic infant male circumcision. Concerned individuals have written

hundreds of letters to public officials such as the federal minister of justice, provincial cabinet ministers, heads of child welfare agencies, and the registrars of colleges of physicians and surgeons in all Canadian jurisdictions. (Nearly 500 such letters are available online.) Unfortunately these authorities are very reluctant even to respond to arguments against routine infant circumcision, much less weigh the facts and provide leadership in eliminating the practice.[112]

After explaining the group's position, a newspaper article quoted a Jewish spokesman to defend circumcision. During extended media coverage of the issue, the only people who defended circumcision were representatives of Jewish or Muslim groups.[113] The lack of any other circumcision advocates suggests that the fear of offending religious groups accounts for the reluctance of Canadian authorities to deal more aggressively with the issue.

Similarly, in Britain, the General Medical Council reviewed the ethics of male circumcision after receiving complaints from the public. They requested and received opinions from various religious organizations, anti-circumcision groups, professional and patients' organizations, and civil rights and children's groups. Religious groups were the only ones to defend the practice.[114-115] Again, it appears that consideration of religious practice limits authorities' responses to the issue.

The effect of religious groups on the practice of non-religious circumcision is noteworthy, considering that they comprise a very small percentage of the population. For example, Jews are only 1.1 percent and Muslims are only two percent of the Canadian population.[116] If the influence of religious groups is that powerful in countries where circumcision is not common, then it appears that this influence needs to be effectively neutralized in order to make progress in circumcision policy at the international level.

9. CONCLUSION

A psychosocial perspective provides a useful framework for examining beliefs and behaviors associated with Jewish circumcision. Empirical findings, emotional conflicts, ethical concerns, and distressing parental experiences are generally ignored by circumcision advocates in favor of religious and spiritual beliefs. If the burden of proof is on those who advocate circumcision, their arguments are not persuasive for questioning non-traditional Jews. Considering the latest information, circumcision cannot be justified based on reason and experience.

According to psychosocial theories, advocating circumcision appears to involve altering experience and beliefs to reduce cognitive inconsistencies and emotional discomfort. Advocates also appear to value messages according to the source of the message and not the content and merits of the message. They are uncritical of religious authorities. Inappropriate charges of anti-Semitism by circumcision advocates call further attention to their avoidance of discussing the merits of circumcision issues. Rather than defensive reaction, the Jewish community would be better served by expanded open debate, particularly with the participation of women.

Jewish and American circumcision are bound in a symbiotic relationship, and there are signs of religious influence that contribute to the perpetuation of circumcision in other English-speaking countries. The existence of religious circumcision in English-speaking countries appears to have a disproportionate inhibiting effect on progressive circumcision policy development.

REFERENCES

1. Soc.culture.jewish.parenting FAQ: Newsgroup Policies and Procedures. URL. http://www.faqs.org/faqs/judaism/FAQ/scjp-admin/.
2. Scott L. The unkindest cut? opponents of circumcision question necessity of Jewish rite. *Jewish Community Voice (NJ)* (August 30, 1995): 9-10.
3. Silverman J. Circumcision: the delicate dilemma. *The Jewish Monthly* (November 1991): 31-35.
4. Sklar J. Breaking with ritual: some Jews believe circumcision causes lingering physical and emotional trauma. *Detroit Jewish News* (March 20, 1998): 67-74.
5. Petty R, Cacioppo J. *Attitudes and Persuasion: Classic and Contemporary Approaches.* Boulder, CO: Westview Press. 1996.
6. Eichner I. Every circumcision is unnecessary. *Yediot* (May 6, 1997): 23. See URL. http://www.kahal.org.
7. Goldman R. Circumcision: a source of Jewish pain. *Jewish Spectator* (Fall, 1997): 16-20.
8. Cohen E. *Guide to Ritual Circumcision and Redemption of the First-Born Son.* New York: Ktav Publishers. 1984: xiii.
9. Kosmin B, Goldstein S, Waksberg J, Lerer N, Keysar A., Scheckner J. *Highlights of the CJF 1990 National Jewish Population Survey.* New York: Council of Jewish Federations. 1991:28.
10. Kosmin B, Goldstein S, Waksberg J, Lerer N, Keysar A., Scheckner J. *Highlights of the CJF 1990 National Jewish Population Survey.* New York: Council of Jewish Federations. 1991:30.
11. Borowitz E. The concept of the covenant in Reform Judaism. In: Barth L, ed. *Berit Milah in the Reform Context.* Berit Milah Board of Reform Judaism. 1990: 155.
12. For a summary of these issues, see Goldman R. *Questioning Circumcision: A Jewish Perspective.* Boston: Vanguard Publications. 1998. Also refer to pertinent chapters in this book.
13. Goldman R. Circumcision: a source of Jewish pain. *Jewish Spectator* (Fall, 1997): 16-20.
14. Kletenik R. It's Brit Milah, not circumcision. *Jewish Spectator* (Winter 1998): 59. All quotes are from the same page.
15. Tam D. In the Greco-Roman arena. *Jewish Spectator* (Winter 1998): 60.

16. For more recent support of sexual and psychological effects, see Boyle G, Goldman R, Svoboda J.S., Fernandez E. Male circumcision: pain, trauma and psychosexual sequelae. *Journal of Health Psychology* 2002;7:329-343.

17. Gordis D. The emotional power of ritual. *Jewish Spectator* (Winter 1998): 61-62.

18. Gordis D. The emotional power of ritual. *Jewish Spectator* (Winter 1998): 61.

19. Gordis D. The emotional power of ritual. *Jewish Spectator* (Winter 1998): 62.

20. Gordis D. The emotional power of ritual. *Jewish Spectator* (Winter 1998): 62.

21. Moss L. Circumcision: a Jewish inquiry. *Midstream.* (January 1992): 20-23.

22. Raul-Friedman E. A rebuttal—circumcision: a Jewish legacy. *Midstream.* (May 1992): 31-33.

23. Raul-Friedman E. A rebuttal—circumcision: a Jewish legacy. *Midstream.* (May 1992): 31-33. [here, p. 31.].

24. Raul-Friedman E. A rebuttal—circumcision: a Jewish legacy. *Midstream.* (May 1992): 31-33. [here, 32.].

25. Raul-Friedman E. A rebuttal—circumcision: a Jewish legacy. *Midstream.* (May 1992): 31-33. [here, 32.].

26. Raul-Friedman E. A rebuttal—circumcision: a Jewish legacy. *Midstream.* (May 1992): 31-33. [here, 33.]. Additional quotes are from the same page.

27. Steinberg M. *Basic Judaism (*rev. ed.) New York: Harcourt Brace Jovanovitch. 1975: 35.

28. Levenson J. The new enemies of circumcision. *Commentary* March 2000: 29-36.

29. Roth J. The meaning for today. *Moment* February 1992: 41-44. [here, p. 43.].

30. American Academy of Pediatrics Task Force on Circumcision. Circumcision policy statement. *Pediatrics* 1999;103:686-693.

31. Australian College of Paediatrics. Position statement: routine circumcision of normal male infants and boys. Parkville, Victoria: Author. 1996.

32. Canadian Paediatric Society. Neonatal circumcision revisited. *Canadian Medical Association Journal* 1996;154:769-780 (Reaffirmed March, 2002). For more recent position statements, see Royal Australasian College of Physicians. Policy statement on circumcision 2002. URL. http://www.racp.edu.au/hpu/paed/circumcision/; British Medical Association. The law and ethics of male circumcision: guidance for doctors 2003. URL. http://www.bma.org.uk/ap.nsf/Content/malecircumcision2003; and American Medical Association. Neonatal circumcision 2000. URL. http://www.ama-assn.org/ama/pub/article/2036-2511.html.

33. American Academy of Pediatrics Task Force on Circumcision. Circumcision policy statement. *Pediatrics* 1999;103:686-693.

34. Levenson J. The new enemies of circumcision. *Commentary* March 2000: 29-36. [here, p. 33.].

35. Goldman R. *Questioning Circumcision: A Jewish Perspective.* Boston: Vanguard Publications. 1998: 63.

36. Compare Levenson, p. 33 with Goldman, p. 61-64.

37. Levenson J. The new enemies of circumcision. *Commentary* March 2000: 29-36. [here, p. 34.].

38. Letters from readers. *Commentary* June 2000: 3-7.

39. Festinger L. *A Theory of Cognitive Dissonance.* Stanford, CA: Stanford University Press. 1957.

40. Festinger L, Carlsmith J. Cognitive consequences of forced compliance. *Journal of Abnormal and Social Psychology* 1959;58:203-210.

41. Beauvois J, Joule R. A radical point of view on dissonance theory. In: Harmon-Jones E, Mills J, eds. *Cognitive Dissonance: Progress on a Pivotal Theory in Social Psychology.* Washington, DC: American Psychological Association. 1999: 43-70.

42. Harmon-Jones E. Toward an understanding of the motivation underlying dissonance: is the production of aversive consequences necessary to produce dissonance? In: Harmon-Jones E, Mills J, eds. *Cognitive Dissonance: Progress on a Pivotal Theory in Social Psychology*. Washington, DC: American Psychological Association. 1999: 71-99.

43. Helfaer P. *The Psychology of Religious Doubt*. Boston: Beacon Press. 1972.

44. Batson C, Schoenrade P, Ventis W. *Religion and the Individual: A Social-Psychological Perspective*. Oxford: Oxford University Press. 1993.

45. Brown L. *The Psychology of Religious Belief*. London: Academic Press. 1987.

46. Raul-Friedman E. letter to the editor. *Midstream* October 1992: 48.

47. Kumpf M, Gotz-Marchand, B. Reduction of cognitive dissonance as a function of magnitude of dissonance, differentiation, and self-esteem. *European Journal of Social Psychology* 1973;3:255-270.

48. Landis D, Robbin S. Gainful pain. *Tikkun* September 1990: 72-74.

49. Gollaher D. *Circumcision: A History of the World's Most Controversial Surgery*. New York: Basic Books. 2000.

50. Goldman R. *Questioning Circumcision: A Jewish Perspective*. Boston: Vanguard Publications. 1998: 15-21.

51. Oswald P, Peltzman P. The cry of the human infant. *Scientific American* 1974;230: 89.

52. Brazelton T. *Doctor and Child*. New York: Delacorte Press. 1976: 31.

53. Call J. quoted in Romberg R. *Circumcision: The Painful Dilemma*. South Hadley, MA: Bergin & Garvey. 1985: 321.

54. Brooks T. quoted in Romberg R. *Circumcision: The Painful Dilemma*. South Hadley, MA: Bergin & Garvey. 1985: 325.

55. Gunnar M, Fisch R., Malone S. The effects of a pacifying stimulus on behavioral and adrenocortical responses to circumcision in the newborn. *Journal of the American Academy of Child Psychiatry* 1984;23:34.

56. Goldman R. *Questioning Circumcision: A Jewish Perspective*. Boston: Vanguard Publications. 1998: 47-52.

57. Hoffman L. *Covenant of Blood*. Chicago: University of Chicago Press. 1996: 218.

58. Rokeach M. *The Open and Closed Mind*. New York: Basic Books. 1960.

59. Freud S. *Psychopathology of Everyday Life*. In: Brill A, ed. and trans. *The Basic Writings of Sigmund Freud*. New York: Modern Library. 1938: 101.

60. Fleiss P. Personal communication. 1994.

61. Romberg R. *Circumcision: The Painful Dilemma*. South Hadley, MA: Bergin & Garvey. 1985: 367.

62. Raynor J, McFarlin D. Motivation and the self-system. In: Sorrentino R, Higgins E, eds. *Handbook of Motivation and Cognition: Foundations of Social Behavior*. New York: Guilford. 1986.

63. Steele C, Liu T. Dissonance processes as self-affirmation. *Journal of Personality and Social Psychology* 1983;45: 5-19.

64. What L. What God takes: bris and mastectomy. *Lilith* Fall 1995: 22-24.

65. Lazarus R, Kanner A, Folkman S. Emotions: a cognitive-phenomenological analysis. In: Plutchick R, Kellerman H, eds. *Emotion: Theory, Research, and Experience*, vol. 1, *Theories of Emotion*. New York: Academic Press. 1980.

66. Walsh M. "Part of Our Tribe": circumcision and Jewish identity. *Burlington (VT) Free Press* (February 5, 1995): 1D, 5D.

67. Foley J. The unkindest cut of all. *Fact* July 1966: 3.

68. Northrup C. Personal communication. 1994.

69. Kunin S, Miller R. The penis becomes a scapegoat. *Moment* December, 1992: 75, 77. See also letters to the editor, *Moment* April 1993: 10-13.

70. Levenson J. The new enemies of circumcision. *Commentary* March 2000: 29-36. [here, p. 34.].
71. Bivas N. Letter to our son's grandparents: why we decided against circumcision. *Humanistic Judaism.* Summer, 1988: 11-13.
72. Moss L. Circumcision: a Jewish inquiry. *Midstream.* January 1992: 20-23.
73. Pollack M. Circumcision: a Jewish feminist perspective. In: Weiner K, Moon A, eds. *Jewish Women Speak Out.* Seattle, WA: Canopy Press. 1995: 171-188.
74. Wallerstein E. *Circumcision: An American Health Fallacy.* New York: Springer Publishing. 1980.
75. Romberg R. *Circumcision: The Painful Dilemma.* South Hadley, MA: Bergin & Garvey. 1985.
76. Whitfield H, ed. BJU International 1999;83(suppl. 1).
77. Denniston G, Hodges F, Milos M, eds. *Male and Female Circumcision: Medical, Legal, and Ethical Considerations in Pediatric Practice.* New York: Kluwer Academic/Plenum Publishers. 1999.
78. Goldman R. *Circumcision: The Hidden Trauma—How an American Cultural Practice Affects Infants and Ultimately Us All.* Boston: Vanguard Publications. 1997: 103-123.
79. Soc.culture.jewish.parenting FAQ: Newsgroup Policies and Procedures. URL. http://www.faqs.org/faqs/judaism/FAQ/scjp-admin/.
80. Frodi A, Lamb M. Sex differences in responsiveness to infants: a developmental study of psychophysical and behavioral responses. *Child Development* 1978;49:1182–8.
81. Bushnell I, Sai F, Mullin J. Neonatal recognition of the mother's face. *British Journal of Developmental Psychology* 1989;7:3-15.
82. DeCasper A, Fifer W. Of human bonding: newborns prefer their mothers' voices. *Science* 1980;208:1174-1176.
83. Pollack M. Circumcision: a Jewish feminist perspective. In: Weiner K, Moon A, eds. *Jewish Women Speak Out.* Seattle, WA: Canopy Press. 1995: 171-188. [here, p. 182.].
84. Goldman R. *Questioning Circumcision: A Jewish Perspective.* Boston: Vanguard Publications. 1998: 55.
85. van der Kolk B. The compulsion to repeat the trauma: re-enactment, revictimization, and masochism. *Psychiatric Clinics of North America* 1989;12:389-411.
86. Goldman R. *Circumcision: The Hidden Trauma—How an American Cultural Practice Affects Infants and Ultimately Us All.* Boston: Vanguard Publications. 1997: 43-45.
87. Stein M, Marx M, Taggert S, Bass R. Routine neonatal circumcision: the gap between contemporary policy and practice. *Journal of Family Practice* 1982;15:47-53.
88. O'Hara K, O'Hara J. The effect of male circumcision on the sexual enjoyment of the female partner. *BJU International* 1999;83(suppl. 1):79-84.
89. Goldman R. *Circumcision: The Hidden Trauma—How an American Cultural Practice Affects Infants and Ultimately Us All.* Boston: Vanguard Publications. 1997: 121-122, 144-148.
90. Goldman R. *Circumcision: The Hidden Trauma—How an American Cultural Practice Affects Infants and Ultimately Us All.* Boston: Vanguard Publications. 1997: 151-153, 162-171. See chapters 4-6 for context of these pages.
91. Bean G, Egelhoff C. Neonatal circumcision: when is the decision made? *Journal of Family Practice* 1984;18:883-887.
92. Ritter T, Denniston G. *Say No To Circumcision.* Aptos, CA: Hourglass. 1996: 16-1.
93. Festinger L. *A Theory of Cognitive Dissonance.* Stanford, CA: Stanford University Press. 1957
94. Greenbaum D, Schonfeld V. The back page: is brit milah cruel and unnecessary? *The Jerusalem Report.* (November 22, 1999):104.

95. Schoen E. The circumcision decision. *Moment* October 1997.

96. Wallerstein E. *Circumcision: An American Health Fallacy.* New York: Springer Publishing. 1980: 154-157.

97. Raul-Friedman E. Circumcision: a Jewish legacy. *Midstream* May 1992:31-33.

98. Levenson J. The new enemies of circumcision. *Commentary* March 2000:29-36.

99. Bailis S. Circumcision: the debate goes on. *Pediatrics* 2000;105:682.

100. Kunin S. Circumcision: the debate goes on. *Pediatrics* 2000;105:683.

101. Shechet J, Tanenbaum B. Circumcision: the debate goes on. *Pediatrics* 2000;105:682-683.

102. Hodges F, Fleiss P. Circumcision: the debate goes on. *Pediatrics* 2000;105:683.

103. Personal communication. 1992.

104. Personal communication. 1992.

105. Howard C, Howard F, Weitzman M. Acetaminophen analgesis in neonatal circumcision: the effect on pain. *Pediatrics* 1994;93:641-646.

106. Personal communication. July 22, 1998.

107. Mahoney L. Personal communication. February 18, 1994.

108. Mahoney L. Personal communication. March 8, 1994.

109. Antonopoulos J. Circumcision: the debate goes on. *Pediatrics* 2000;105:684.

110. Rickwood A, Kenny S, Donnell S. Towards evidence based circumcision of English boys: survey of trends in practice. *British Medical Journal* 2000;321:792-793.

111. Humphreys A. Circumcision is against the charter, group says. *National Post* (February 12, 2001:Sect. A1.

112. Association for Genital Integrity. Court challenge: a strategic approach to ending infant male circumcision. URL. http://www.courtchallenge.com/main/overvw1.html.

113. Bhimji A. Personal communication. February 2001.

114. General Medical Council. Guidance for doctors who are asked to circumcise male children. London: General Medical Council.

115. Beecham L. GMC issues guidelines on circumcision. British Medical Journal, 1997;314:1573.

116. Statistics Canada. Canadian statistics: selected religions, provinces and territories. URL. http://www.statcan.ca/english/Pgdb/demo30a.htm. 2001.

Chapter 14

MY PAINFUL JOURNEY
A Retired Jewish Physician's Acknowledgment of Circumcision Trauma Leads Him to Activism

Mark D. Reiss, MD
Vice President, Doctors Opposing Circumcision (DOC)

Abstract: Most men who are circumcised in infancy live their lives with no conscious memory or regret of their own trauma. As a result, they are frequently inaccessible for dialogue. Denying any injury, they tend to inflict their sons in similar fashion, aided and abetted in the United States by the mythologies of medicine. In Judaism, this is especially problematical, because of longstanding custom and tradition based on the biblical covenant. The personal history of a Jewish physician's recognition, at the age of sixty-five, of his own infant circumcision trauma, is recounted. The considerable psychic pain endured by this discovery leads to further conflicts within his family, the medical community, and his own Jewish congregation, when he begins to speak out against circumcision. After a few short years, he has now joined the ranks of human rights advocates.

Keywords: Circumcision, Jewish ritual, Judaism, trauma

1.   INTRODUCTION

When I think of what I want to say about how the subject of circumcision has influenced my life, two questions come to mind, aside from the question, "Why was I circumcised in the first place?" They both begin with the word *why*.

Why might it be of interest to chronicle my story? After all, many men before me have described dissatisfaction, anger, remorse and pain relating to their infant circumcision. Their reports have been widely circulated in various publications, one example being in the *Men's Voices...* columns of Jim Bigelow's *The Joy of Uncircumcising!*[1] There have been other

Flesh and Blood, Edited by Denniston et al.
Kluwer Academic/Plenum Publishers, New York 2004

physicians, other Jews, others in the sixty-year old age group who have spoken and written of their feelings. Some of these men have become active in the movement to end circumcision. So why is my story special? Maybe one satisfactory answer is that if I, a sixty-five-year-old Jewish physician, could suddenly recognize my circumcision trauma, and within three short years start to make changes in my life and also in others' lives, then this could happen to anyone.

Why did this "awakening" happen to me? At times, in moments of depression and anguish, I have even asked myself, "Why did this *have to* happen to me?" I was happy in my ignorance. Why couldn't I have just remained in that complacent cocoon, unconscious of my infantile trauma? Why was I not spared the anguish of that discovery? I hardly ask that question today. Although frustration and sadness seem to be repetitive themes in this work, my feelings about human rights activism have in general been very positive. In large part this is directly related to the many wonderful and caring people I have met and worked with, who share my enthusiasm in contemplating a world free of circumcision.

2.   PRIOR TO RECOGNITION OF CIRCUMCISION TRAUMA

I grew up in a middle class Jewish home with a large extended family. Ritual circumcision (*brit [or bris] milah*) was a common family event. Later, in medical school, I saw and even participated in circumcisions. Although mildly uncomfortable with the procedure, I never considered questioning circumcision, and when my son was born, there was no doubt that he would have a *bris*. I have a vague memory in the 1960s of reading an article entitled *The Rape of the Phallus*,[2] which caused a figurative rise of my eyebrows, but nothing more at the time. However, the article must have affected me subliminally; otherwise, why would I remember it from so many years ago?

I was leading a good life, had a wonderfully fulfilled marriage, raised two great children who each were now happily married, and my successful career in medicine had voluntarily ended in early retirement with ample time now to pursue my love of piano performance. My active and vigorous sex life was undiminished. Life was good. I had no reason to believe that a major trauma had befallen me when I was an infant. Until I was sixty-five years old, when several quite remarkable things happened to me, almost in serendipitous fashion.

3.   RECOGNITION OF TRAUMA

In March of 1999, two dramatic events were taking place in my family. My beloved father-in-law, almost ninety years of age, was dying. He was the last of the older generation, and my own concerns of mortality were ripe. At the same time, I learned that both of my children were expecting their first child. I was simultaneously about to become a first time grandfather and the newest member of the older generation. Perhaps when we contemplate the beginnings and ends of life, intuitive senses are sharpened. I don't know. But it seems to me now, that it was inevitable that the light bulb was about to be turned on.

I have for several years indulged myself in a weekly massage. My massage therapist is also trained in the Rosen Method,[3] and would frequently utilize this subtle touch therapy towards the end of my massage, during which time I would fall into a deep reverie. I remember feeling very fragile and vulnerable at those times, almost infantile. My Rosen Method practitioner had remarked to me that this type of behavior could indicate childhood trauma, and that it is not uncommon for clients to become aware of incidents of sexual abuse during therapy. At one of these sessions, I noted a deep pain in my genital area, and my hands involuntarily moved to protect myself. I began to cry and was very disturbed. The session soon ended, and when we spoke of what had happened, I was questioned about any memories of childhood abuse or injury in my genital area. The possibility was raised of circumcision being the source of my remembered pain. I denied any knowledge or recognition of pain relating to my circumcision. I simply could not accept the fact that a profound trauma locked in my body and brain had been released by this therapy. I might have again repressed the pain, but luckily the information gap in my knowledge was soon to be corrected.

Five days later, while on a bicycle trip, my wife and I stopped at a coffee shop. There were some dog-eared books for sale on a table in a corner of the shop. My eyes were drawn to one entitled *Questioning Circumcision: A Jewish Perspective.*[4] As I picked up the book and started reading, I was flooded with immediate recollection about what had happened at my massage. I bought the book, which luckily just fit in a pocket of my bike shirt. That evening I voraciously read the entire book at one sitting. I slept poorly that night and the next day again studied the book. Its message resonated deeply within my body, and I was shaken to the core.

I can only describe the next few months as a period of intense anxiety and mourning for my lost foreskin. My sexual experiences in life had been so very important to me, and I now felt cheated, robbed of sensations that I would never know. Raging anger and uncontrolled sobbing were daily occurrences. I was totally obsessed with the topic of circumcision. I studied websites, read voraciously, and viewed videos on the subject. Although I was starting on a primitive path to activism, the going was rough and rocky. I was so keenly focused on my own pain that I could not understand why my feelings were not uniformly embraced and accepted by everyone with whom I spoke. Moreover, my knowledge was far too sketchy for me to be an effective lobbyist against circumcision.

Even during the earliest expressions of grief, my wife was very supportive. She could not completely understand the depth of my feelings but she was always present for me. However, her advice to control myself during discussions with others was unfortunately not followed, and my over-zealous approach produced uniformly bad results. During this time period there were several painful interactions with family members. I believe that the wounds from those early arguments have largely healed, but some scars probably will always linger.

I have learned from those experiences that a cool and dispassionate tone, and presentation of facts in a clear and concise form is always best when discussing circumcision. An aggressive posture, and use of inflammatory phrases such as *barbaric custom, genital mutilation* will be counterproductive, especially when speaking with people who are just beginning to have their consciousness raised on the subject. They will simply stop listening. Nevertheless, I still occasionally find myself slipping back into "zealous mode," and I always regret it.

4.   HELP FROM THE ACTIVIST COMMUNITY

The day after reading Ronald Goldman's book, phone contact with Goldman led me to Tim Hammond, who lives only a few minutes walk from my home. In addition to supplying me with a copy of his video *Whose Body, Whose Rights?*,[5] Tim saw that I was going through a difficult time and graciously spent a few hours talking with me. From Tim, I was referred to a Bay Area Activist meeting, which was scheduled for that very weekend. I attended the meeting and was welcomed with open arms. The group was incredibly empathetic and patiently listened to my story. The meeting essentially turned into a group therapy session for me. I immediately saw that I had a community with whom I would have continuing contact. Many of the individuals that I met for the first time that afternoon have been extremely influential in my developing activism.

5.   TEACHING MEDICAL STUDENTS

One of the women at that meeting was Norma Wilcox. We became close friends and when Norma asked me to join a group of men who were teaching physical examination of the male genital tract to sophomore medical students, I gladly agreed. These talented and dedicated men (a group of women also work with the students, instructing them in gynecologic examinations) are a diverse group. Some are body workers, nurses, sex therapists and psychologists. I am the only physician currently in this group of teaching associates. For the past twenty years, Norma has been coordinating this incredibly successful program in the Bay Area, for University of California at San Francisco (UCSF) and Stanford Medical School, and Touro School of Osteopathy.

Each instructor spends three hours with a small group of students (typically three) exploring the details of how to carefully, respectfully, and gently examine the male genitalia, and how to speak with patients about sexual matters. We instructors also serve as models, and we demonstrate our own anatomy, and then have the students examine us. Of course, their medical faculty trains the students as well, but our instruction goes beyond the traditional medical curriculum. This technique has been recommended as an excellent method of teaching medical students in an area otherwise considered problematical.[6]

I immediately saw this as an opportunity to talk to these fledgling physicians about medical circumcision, and show them why we need to stop routine infant circumcision in the United States. Although genital integrity is not the primary focus of these training sessions, I know that all the instructors speak about circumcision, and therefore the entire medical student body in the Bay Area is getting some instruction about genital integrity. I, personally, made it a very high priority in my teaching, spending about thirty minutes on the subject. For every young physician I successfully interacted with, just think of the number of foreskins that can be saved over the course of that physician's career! I was involved in the program for three years, and have had contact with about fifty student physicians.

6.   OTHER MEDICAL ACTIVITIES

I have joined Dr. Morris Sorrells as one of the physician researchers in a *Penile Sensitivity Touch-Test Evaluation.*[7] I look forward to the results of our study adding to the body of medical literature showing the foreskin's unique role in the sensation of the penis.

At the recent American Academy of Pediatrics (AAP) meeting in San Francisco, I carried a placard reading: JEWISH PHYSICIAN OPPOSING CIRCUMCISION. I received a number of "thumbs up" and smiles. One physician stopped to chat, looking for ways to respond to parents who demanded circumcision. I think I offered him some positive suggestions. However, more people either looked away, or actually scowled at me. A number of physicians stopped and berated me. Two of these were Jewish and quite irate. One Muslim pediatrician almost threatened physical harm in his anger. But the longest and most offensive diatribe came from an Evangelical Christian man who, quoting biblical chapter and verse, kept me busy for about fifteen minutes. This experience in the activist trenches gave me a painful taste of the challenges we face in the medical community.

7.   EFFORTS WITHIN JUDAISM

Very early in the evolution of my knowledge about circumcision, I knew that my primary focus would be in my own religion. I realized that as a practicing Jew, I could better challenge circumcision from within. I wanted very much to speak out in my own Conservative congregation. But I was insecure about my knowledge on the subject, and fearful of rejection by my fellow congregants.

Circumcision is not an identity issue in religious laws of Judaism. However, in the minds of many Jews, keeping the biblical tradition of this ritual of God's covenant with Israel is tantamount to the very ethos of being Jewish. In years past, Jews have been martyred rather than give up circumcision. During the holocaust, newborn boys were circumcised in the cattle cars on the way to crematoria. It is a very highly charged subject, and therefore challenging Jewish circumcision cannot be taken lightly. So, of course I was worried about coming out publicly in my own Jewish community.

Our rabbi is very approachable, and I have a good relationship with him, and so, a few months after the initial recognition of my own circumcision trauma, I met with him. It was a pleasant, non-confrontational interaction, and I left the meeting feeling pleased that I had made the effort. Shortly after this, he announced to me that when a reporter from a Jewish newspaper on the East Coast had called asking him about a perceived movement within Conservative Judaism questioning circumcision, he gave the reporter my name and phone number as a contact. This information elicited some minor panic, since I did not think I knew enough to speak publicly, and moreover I wanted no part of being a spokesperson for this "movement." A crash course on circumcision ensued, but luckily the reporter never called.

I had been talking privately with a number of my friends in the congregation who I thought would support my right to speak out against circumcision. I was gratified by some confidential information from a few of them who actually told me that they agreed with my position. Those, who, although disagreeing with my position, supported my right to speak out, fortified me in my desire to speak to the entire congregation. Of course I did not speak with any of the more reactionary congregants; I would deal with them later.

It took me more than a year from that first talk with my rabbi to summon up the courage to put something out on our congregational community e-mail list. I called it *Circumcision...My Position.*[8]

After this first posting, I got some negative comments, but I felt that I had not covered the issue of sexuality sufficiently, and so I sent a second notice to our list. This created quite a furor. It was then that I first fully understood Leonard Glick's statement "...question[ing] infant male circumcision before a Jewish audience...is not a path to popularity."[9] I was called a "heretic"[1] and my positions as an officer in the synagogue, director, and chair of a major committee were challenged. I was asked to stop talking about circumcision, but I have refused to comply with this request. Now, whenever I post an item, I insert a disclaimer that the statements represent my personal opinion only, and do not reflect either synagogue policy, or bear any relationship to my positions within the congregation.

I have given up on my original plan to organize a discussion on the topic in the setting of my Conservative synagogue. Perhaps a Reform temple might be interested in sponsoring such a forum? I am also investigating the possibility of a detailed discussion group in the setting of a Renewal movement summer program.

When an extensive article on Ritual Circumcision (*brit milah*) appeared in our local newspaper,[10] I wrote a letter to the editor (which they printed) stating that not all Jews circumcise[11] and spoke of *brit shalom*, or non-cutting naming ceremony similar to that used for baby girls.

This got me thinking of all the parents who may wish to speak to rabbis or other experienced lay leaders who could officiate at such a ceremony, or help them devise their own ceremony. I now have a web-page entitled "Celebrants of Brit Shalom" which has been incorporated into Hugh Young's excellent www.circumstitions.com website. My page can be accessed at:

http://www.circumstitions.com/Jewish-shalom.html

ı One of my rabbi's most endearing comments to me was when he said, with a twinkle in his eye, "Of course you are a heretic, Mark...but I love heretics!"

At latest count, we list twenty-seven celebrants in the United States, and recently have listed celebrants internationally, in United Kingdom, Canada, and Israel.

Through these efforts I have already successfully introduced numerous prospective parents wishing to have non-cutting ceremonies to individuals who can help them. Hardly a week goes by that I do not get one or several such requests.

It is claimed that only forty percent of newborn Jewish boys in Sweden are now being circumcised.[12] This figure is quite astounding, compared with other countries. Although the number of Jews in Sweden is relatively small (20,000), one cannot dismiss the fact that if a country or community strongly denounces circumcision (as Sweden has done) it can affect the Jewish population of this community in their practice of circumcision.

8.   RESTORATION

In October 2001, I made the decision to join the more than twenty-thousand men throughout the world[13] who are attempting restoration of their foreskins. Within a few short months I had achieved a measure of success, so that, when I asked one group of medical students, "What do you see," pointing to my penis, they *all* responded, "Well...uh...you haven't been circumcised!"

This not only gave me a chuckle, but also has been decidedly therapeutic.

I am continuing the restoration process.

9.   CONCLUSION

All men circumcised in infancy have been traumatized, but it is difficult to convince adult men of this fact. It almost takes a revelation, an epiphany, a leap of insight to close the gap of ignorance, fear, and repressed trauma, to enable us to come to realize and admit the harm of our own circumcision. I was fortunate enough to have been given that insight. As it was, I needed both emotional and intellectual catalysts to fully understand my own trauma. I am firmly convinced that one of our most important goals is to help others achieve that same insight. Our strongest weapon against those who would perpetuate circumcision in the United States is that we have the facts. We must continue to provide the physicians and lay population of the United States with the kinds of reliable information that have been the hallmark of our movement. As the general public and our physicians are gaining more awareness of the harms of circumcision, the numbers of "prophylactic" infant circumcisions in the United States are slowly dropping, especially on the West Coast. I may be a naïve optimist. However, I hope to be able to see the end of routine medical circumcision in the United States within my own lifetime.

Once medical circumcision ends in our country, many of the assimilated and unaffiliated Jewish Americans, now having their boys circumcised in the hospitals, will likely follow the lead and stop having their infants circumcised. However, with the affiliated and observant Jewish population, covenantal tradition and longstanding customs firmly reign. Even though more and more young Jewish couples are now having discussions about possibly not circumcising, only a few actually make that choice. It is not likely that official laws of circumcision will change within the religion in the near future. This was attempted before,[14] in Frankfurt, Germany in 1843, but was not successful. We Jews have been circumcising our newborn boys for approximately 2,500 years. It may take another 2,500 years to completely end circumcision in Judaism. We are a patient people, and with time, maybe, just maybe, it might happen.

10.   ACKNOWLEDGMENTS

Numerous individuals have helped me to endure the initial pain experienced following recognition of my circumcision trauma, and have shown me the road to help others through activism. I am deeply grateful to all of you.

The gentle hands of Elyze Stewart, my Rosen Method practitioner, were the catalysts for the first perception of my infantile trauma, and for that I owe Elyze a profound debt. I would like to thank Lisa Braver Moss, a freelance writer who has written extensively in opposition to circumcision in Judaism, for her help in editing this paper. Tim Hammond was thankfully present early in my painful journey, and kindly guided me to others who could be of aid to me. To Norma Wilcox, who aided me immeasurably with early therapeutic efforts, and introduced me to the medical students, my thanks. Wayne Griffiths, Co-founder and Executive Director of National Organization of Restoring Men (NORM) has been my personal trainer and guru in the quest for restoration of my own foreskin; many thanks for your patience and help. I am deeply grateful to the creative and cooperative web-meister of my "Celebrants of Brit Shalom" web-page, Hugh Young. And what can I say to Marilyn Milos, the *Mother of Us All*...where would we be, but for you?

Finally, with enduring love, I want to thank my wife Joan Reinhardt Reiss, whose incredible support and wise counsel has enabled me to stay on course throughout this remarkable journey.

REFERENCES

1. Bigelow J. The Joy of Uncircumcising! (2nd edition). Aptos: California: Hourglass Publishers, 1995.
2. Morgan WKC. The rape of the phallus. JAMA 1965;193:223-4.
3. Mayland EL. Rosen Method: An approach to wholeness and well-being through the body. Palo Alto, California: Elaine Loomis Mayland; 1984. (Eleventh Printing, 2000).
4. Goldman R. Questioning Circumcision: A Jewish Perspective. Boston: Vanguard Publications, 1998.
5. Hammond T (Executive Producer), Dillon L (Director). Whose Body, Whose Rights? (Video). San Francisco: Dillonwood Productions; 1995.
6. Robins LS, Alexander GL, Dicken LL, Belville WD, Zweifler AJ. The effect of a standardized patient instructor experience on students' anxiety and confidence levels performing the male genitorectal examination. Teaching and Learning in Medicine 1997;9:264-9.
7. Sorrells M. Penile Sensitivity Touch-Test Evaluation Study. Delivered at The Seventh International Symposium on Human Rights and Modern Society: Advancing Human dignity and the Legal Right to Bodily Integrity in the 21st Century. Washington, D.C.; 2002.
8. Reiss MD. Circumcision...My Position. September, 2001. (Revised 2002). See Appendix. Also see National Organization of Circumcision Information Resource Centers (NOCIRC) web page: <http://www.nocirc.org/>
9. Glick LB. Jewish Circumcision: An enigma in historical perspective. In: Denniston GC, Hodges FM, Milos MF, editors. Understanding Circumcision: A multi-disciplinary approach to a multi-dimensional problem. New York: Plenum Publishers; 2001. 19-20.
10. McManis S. Jewish bris ceremony shows you're never too young for tradition. San Francisco Chronicle, Living section: page E1; Sunday, 30 December 2001.
11. Reiss MD. Letters to the Editor, San Francisco Chronicle, Living section (Sunday, January 6, 2002). p. E2.
12. Personal communication from Yngve Hofvander who cites: Abramowics L, Carlberg A, Posner-Körösi L. Blir manlig omskärelse förbjuden om 4 år. (Will circumcision in males be forbidden in 4 years?). Lakartidningen (Official Journal for the Swed Med Assoc) nr 36, 2001; 98: 3835-6. Using the figure of 20,000 Jews in Sweden, and assuming that the birth rate in Jews is the same as in the general population (10 per 1,000), 100 Jewish boys would be born in Sweden every year. Since only 40 infant Jewish circumcisions are registered (all circumcisions must be registered with the government), that would = 40 %.
13. Personal communication from R. Wayne Griffiths, Co-founder and Executive Director of National Organization of Restoring Men (NORM).
14. Hoffman LA. Covenant of Blood: Circumcision and Gender in Rabbinic Judaism. Chicago: The University of Chicago Press; 1996. 2-9.

APPENDIX

CIRCUMCISION: MY POSITION

Mark D. Reiss, M.D. (revised 2002)

I am a sixty-nine-year-old retired physician, a Jew who is an active member of a Conservative synagogue, and a grandfather.

When I was in Medical School in the 1950s, almost all newborn males were circumcised. Despite the fact that prophylactic surgery was not generally performed, we were taught that circumcision was the correct and healthy thing to do. It was thought to control masturbation, decrease cancer risk, and help curtail sexually transmitted diseases. We learned nothing of foreskin anatomy and function. Infant nervous systems were thought to be undeveloped and their pain was so trivialized that it was almost ignored. As a young physician, I participated in many circumcisions. Over the years I've witnessed *brit milah* in the homes of friends and family. I was mildly uncomfortable with the practice, but like most physicians, and like most Jews, I said and did nothing to question circumcision.

Three years ago, as I was about to become a grandfather for the first time, my interest in the subject became more focused. I learned that more and more physicians now realize that any potential benefits of circumcision are far outweighed by its risks and drawbacks. The American Academy of Pediatrics has stated that "Routine circumcision is not necessary." Whether done by a physician in the hospital, or a *mohel* in a ritual *brit milah*, the procedure has significant complication rates of infection, hemorrhage and even death. Mortality may actually be higher than thought since some of these deaths have not been attributed to circumcision, but listed only under their secondary causes, such as hemorrhage or infection. I've learned of the very important role the foreskin has in the protection of the head of the penis in the infant, and in sexual functioning in adulthood. It has also been shown that the newborn feels pain even more acutely than adults do, and that many of the infants who stop crying during circumcision are actually in a state of traumatic shock. To my amazement I learned that the USA is now the *only* country in the world routinely circumcising newborn babies for non-religious reasons.

With these overwhelming reasons not to circumcise, I began to look at the practice of ritual circumcision in the Jewish community and I learned that: circumcision is *not* an identity issue. You do not *need* to be circumcised to be Jewish any more than the need to observe many other Jewish laws. The bottom line is this: if your mother is Jewish, you are Jewish, period. And in the Reform tradition, patrilineal descent is also accepted. Among Jews in Europe, (only forty percent of newborn Jewish boys in Sweden are being circumcised) South America, and even in Israel, circumcision is not universal. Growing numbers of American Jews are now leaving their sons intact as they view circumcision as a part of Jewish law that they can no longer accept. Alternative *brit b'li milah* or *brit shalom* ceremonies (ritual naming ceremony without cutting) are being performed by some rabbis. Increasing numbers of intact boys are going to religious school, having *bar mitzvahs*, and taking their place as young adults in the Jewish community.

As a Jewish grandfather, I want to assure young couples about to bring a child into the world, that there are other members of the Jewish "older" generation, including other Jewish physicians, and even some rabbis, who feel as I do. If your heart and instincts tell you to leave your son intact, listen!

Chapter 15

NORTH CAROLINA MEDICAID AND THE FUNDING OF ROUTINE NON-THERAPEUTIC CIRCUMCISIONS

Amber Craig, MA
Director, National Organization of Circumcision Information Resouce Centers of North Carolina

Abstract: There is growing sentiment across the United States that tax dollars should not be wasted on medically unnecessary circumcisions. Bills have been introduced in California, Florida, Mississippi, Missouri, Montana, Nevada, New Mexico, North Dakota, Oregon, Utah, Washington, as well as some private HMOs serving Oklahoma's Medicaid recipients, to eliminate Medicaid funding of elective circumcision. This paper focuses on the successful efforts of citizens of North Carolina to lobby the state legislature to eliminate Medicaid funding for routine infant circumcision and instead provide for only the medically necessary needs of its state residents.

Key words: Medicaid, circumcision

1.   INTRODUCTION

Effective 1 November 2001, North Carolina Medicaid suspended payments for routine circumcision. This policy change was announced to all North Carolina physicians in October 2001 through the state Medicaid bulletin by stating "The American Academy of Pediatrics (AAP) policy on circumcision states that the benefits are not significant enough for the AAP to recommend circumcision as a routine procedure"[1]

The practice of routinely circumcising male babies is not recommended or endorsed by any national or international medical organization in the world. The American Medical Association,[2] the American Academy of

Pediatrics,[3] and the American College of Obstetrics and Gynecology[4] consider routine circumcision of male infants to be a medically unnecessary procedure performed for cosmetic, social, or religious reasons, and these organizations do not recommend it as a routine medical procedure.

Worldwide, circumcision of the male or female genitals is rare. Routine circumcision is not performed in Europe, Australia, most of Asia, Latin America, or in South America. Eighty-five percent of the world's male population and ninety-eight percent of the world's female population are not circumcised.[5]

The North Carolina legislative action was part of a growing movement across the nation against tax dollar funding of medically unnecessary circumcisions. Six state Medicaid agencies, California, North Dakota, Oregon, Washington, Nevada, and Mississippi, as well as some private HMOs serving Oklahoma's Medicaid recipients have already suspended coverage for optional circumcisions.[6] In spring of 2001, the Michigan Legislature began debating a bill to end Medicaid circumcision funding, the status of that bill is still pending.[7]

2.   INITIAL MEDIA AND MEDICAL ESTABLISHMENT REACTION

When the new circumcision policy was announced, a handful of North Carolina physicians began pressuring the North Carolina Legislature to reinstate circumcision funding.[8-9] A state newspaper profiled these physicians' effort to alert the North Carolina Legislature about their discontent. On 31 October 2001, the *Raleigh News and Observer* ran a front-page news story titled "Medicaid won't cover circumcision" detailing complaints from doctors upset about this policy change.[10] The article detailed plans state physicians were undertaking to reverse the policy of not funding routine non-therapeutic circumcision. According to the article, Valerie Parisi, MD, chair of the OB/GYN Department at University of North Carolina Hospital, held discussions with the heads of the large hospitals and medical schools within North Carolina to create a position paper advocating that the North Carolina Legislature reinstate elective circumcision funding.[11] William Hubbard, MD, President of the North Carolina Pediatric Society, was quoted in the same article as saying, "As advocates for children, the North Carolina Pediatric Society would like Medicaid families to have the same choices for children that everybody else has."[12] This position is confounding given his recent statement published in January's Governing Magazine in which Hubbard declares, "We don't advocate circumcision as a medical necessity."[13] The *News and Observer* article reported on the position of doctors upset over loss of non-medical circumcision funding, yet it did not interview anyone that supported the policy change. The reporter and her editor were contacted by several individuals that requested the *News and Observer* interview North Carolina citizens that supported this new policy. The editor hung up on Dr. Kenneth Baker, a practicing North Carolina obstetrician and expert on the foreskin and circumcision, when he requested equal press coverage regarding why many North Carolinians supported the state not covering elective circumcision.[14] During this same time period, no other major newspaper in North Carolina covered this story.

3. ECONOMIC INCENTIVE FOR MAINTAINING ROUTINE CIRCUMCISION

United States Medicaid finances over twenty-five percent of all infant circumcisions nationwide.[15] In North Carolina, one out of every two pregnant women receives Medicaid assistance.[16] North Carolina physicians earn more to perform unnecessary circumcisions on Medicaid babies than physicians in almost every other state in the nation. In the year 2000, North Carolina Medicaid paid physicians $166 for elective circumcision, nearly double the US Medicaid average of $85.19.[17] Most other states pay substantially less. New York reimbursed only $12, New Jersey $16, Maryland $18, Colorado $38.11, and Texas $50.75 in 2000.[18] In 1999, North Carolina Medicaid spent more on unnecessary circumcision than almost every state in the nation.[19] For calendar year 2000, North Carolina Medicaid wasted $1.8 million dollars funding elective circumcisions.[20] Longer hospital stays that result from circumcision also add to the total Medicaid costs. Professor Christopher J. Mansfield of the East Carolina University School of Medicine conducted a study of cost factors and the length of hospital stay associated with routine male circumcision. Professor Mansfield and colleagues reported that, when an infant is scheduled for circumcision, both mother and child remain in the hospital an average of six hours longer than they would if no circumcision were scheduled. Professor Mansfield reports that, during this time, both mother and baby consume large and expensive hospital services including room, board, nursing services, nursery care, and other services.[21] Professor Mansfield and colleagues estimate that the longer stay by each mother and child for circumcision adds $900 per day to the total hospital bill in 1990-91 dollars. Therefore, 0.26 day multiplied by $900 equals $234.00 in increased hospital costs per circumcised child in addition to the actual circumcision fee.[22]

A recent study in *Pediatrics* concluded that physicians significantly under-informed parents regarding the risks and benefits of routine non-therapeutic circumcision.[23] This study found that nine out of ten parents were not given adequate information, and some male infants are being circumcised without parental consent or knowledge. This is especially true for economically or educationally disadvantaged parents. The American Academy of Pediatrics stresses in their current 1999 policy statement that "Physicians counseling families concerning this decision should assist parents by explaining potential benefits and risks, and by ensuring that they understand circumcision is an elective procedure."[24]

4.   CONTINUED MEDIA PRESSURE

The media pressure on the North Carolina Legislature to reinstate funding continued with an opinion column by Ruth Sheehan that ran in the *Raleigh News and Observer* on 5 November 2001 titled "Save $200 and Shame a Poor Boy." Ms. Sheehan laments that, "...thanks to North Carolina state lawmakers (many of whom ought to be minding their own zippers, thanks), boys born to mothers receiving Medicaid will no longer be circumcised with state dollars. Instead they will be marked with the scarlet P; or U (for uncircumcised)."[25] Ms. Sheehan's commentary is not supported by current national statistics on infant circumcision showing that nearly half of American parents in 1999 chose to protect their newborn sons from circumcision, and over sixty percent of parents on the West Coast decline this elective procedure.[26]

During the month of November, the *News and Observer* printed ten letters to the editor responding to their coverage of circumcision; not one letter supported reinstatement of tax funding for unnecessary circumcisions.

5.   LEGISLATIVE ACTION TO APPEASE DOCTORS

The North Carolina House added funding for "optional" circumcisions to Senate Bill 841, a bill with numerous other unrelated clauses, and passed it on 16 November 2001. North Carolina Representative David Redwine, co-chairman of the House Appropriations Committee, was quoted by the *News and Observer* as saying, "That cut will be restored, if you'll pardon the description."[27] After the House passed Bill 841, the bill then went to the North Carolina Senate for approval.

6. GRASSROOTS EFFORTS AND LEGISLATIVE SUPPORT BUILDS

As North Carolina taxpayers, concerned parents, and citizens became aware of the legislative attempt to restore optional circumcision funding, they launched into action — telephoning, e-mailing, and writing the senators with their concerns. Legislators reported being overwhelmed by hundreds of contacts.[28-30]

In the final days of the legislative session, North Carolina citizens were receiving very encouraging news from the senators. Senate Appropriations Chairs Odom and Forrester, as well as committee member Senator Moore all expressed strong support in e-mails to constituents and indicated that the Senate would not pass the reinstatement of funding by the House.[31-33]

7. THE GOVERNOR GETS INVOLVED AND FUNDING IS REINSTATED

In the final days, however, many senators also started reporting that the pressure to keep circumcision funding was coming from the Governor's office.[34]

No action had been taken on SB 841 by the final day of the legislative session, 6 December 2001. It appeared no action would be taken on this bill before the session ended. During the final hours of the session some key senators on the appropriations committee in the senate had already gone home. The final voting record shows that fifteen of the fifty senators were not present for the vote.[35] In last minute budget negotiations, Section twelve reinstating funding for optional circumcisions was taken out of Senate Bill 841 and added to House Bill 231, becoming section nineteen.[36] This bill was then approved by the Legislature along with numerous other bills before officially adjourning. HB 231 was long, and considering that legislators were giving approval to numerous bills in the session's final hours, it is unclear how many of the legislators knew that optional circumcision funding had been added to the bill. The final voting record shows only twenty-three of fifty senators voted in favor of HB 231, and of these senators, some informed constituents that they did not support the circumcision clause even though they voted for the overall bill.[37-39] In the House, seventy-eight of the one-hundred-twenty representatives voted for the overall bill.[40]

Franklin Freeman, a close aide to Governor Michael Easley, reported that the Governor went out of his way to make sure circumcision funding got reinstated because he did not want Medicaid children to be marked as poor.

Freeman admitted the Governor also received guidance and counseling from his brother, an obstetrician practicing in North Carolina.[41]

8.   CONTINUED MEDIA BIAS

Governing Magazine continued the media distortions of the North Carolina Medicaid controversy in their January 2002 issue. Despite the small number of legislators in favor of circumcision funding, *Governing Magazine* reports, "The legislature abruptly changed course and voted overwhelmingly to restore funding."[42]

Donna Larkin is a North Carolina mother with three children who recently were added to a state sponsored health insurance program, but beforehand had no health insurance at all. Larkin's children had been on a state waiting list for almost a year before they were able to acquire the state sponsored insurance. Larkin, a grocery store clerk, and her disabled husband continue to be without any medical insurance. She objected to non-medical circumcision funding with her tax dollars when her own family could not receive assistance for basic medical needs. Larkin contacted the *News and Observer* and asked the paper to write a story about her situation and the North Carolina taxpayer's perspective of this issue, but they declined, saying they felt the paper had already covered enough of this circumcision story.[43] Donna also called the *Raleigh Associated Press* and some other North Carolina newspapers, but they did not feel people were upset about taxpayer funding of non-medical procedures.

9.   THE CONCLUSION OF THE 2001 LEGISLATIVE SESSION

Following the conclusion of the 2001 legislative session, the President Pro Tempore of the North Carolina General Assembly, Marc Basnight, sent a letter to all North Carolina citizens who contacted him about this issue. He states, "While I understand there is debate in the medical community about the merits of circumcision, I supported this legislation because I believe it is important, when possible, to allow Medicaid patients the same choice for care that patients with private medical insurance receive....My hope is that the General Assembly's action on this issue will allow parents of Medicaid-eligible children will [sic] make the decision about circumcision the same way those parents with private insurance do: by discussing the procedure with their family doctor and making a rational, informed decision about which option best reflects their values."[44]

While making circumcision funding a budget priority, the Legislature failed to provide for the medical needs of the state's poor and disabled citizens. Despite a current lawsuit, the General Assembly failed to allocate the money needed to provide adequate dental care to the state's 672,000 poor children struggling to get this care. Currently Medicaid children in forty of the state's counties have no access to any private dentist because the reimbursement rates for dental care are deplorably low.[45] The state's impoverished disabled elderly citizens also did not fare well at the conclusion of the legislative session. Budget cuts froze the program that offers in-home assistance to elderly poor who qualify. According to an article in the *News and Observer*, "Advocates for the elderly say state Medicaid officials took the easy way out and should have trimmed other Medicaid services instead of completely freezing the one for the disabled elderly."[46]

10.   THE FUTURE OF THE MEDICAID BATTLE IN NORTH CAROLINA

North Carolina is currently experiencing a budget deficit of at least $900 million dollars. Governor Easley has issued a seven percent budget cut.[47] Medicaid currently accounts for thirteen percent of the total General Fund budget in North Carolina, and traditionally has shown a fifteen percent annual growth rate.[48] The state Medicaid program is currently facing a $108 million budget shortfall.[49] The North Carolina Legislature reconvenes in May 2002, but the appropriations leaders will most likely return earlier to work on the budget crisis. It is predicted that severe cuts to Medicaid will need to be part of a feasible budget.[50]

There is growing sentiment across the nation that tax dollars should not be wasted on medically unnecessary circumcisions. In addition to the legislative actions in North Carolina during the past year, bills have been introduced in Missouri, Michigan, and New Mexico to eliminate elective circumcision funding through Medicaid. Given the waning popularity of elective circumcision and the pressure on North Carolina to reduce unnecessary expenditures, North Carolina citizens opposed to tax dollar funding of non-medical circumcision hope North Carolina will soon join other states in recognizing that tax dollars should not fund optional cultural circumcisions, and instead provide for only the medically necessary needs of its state residents.

11.   ADDENDUM, SUMMER 2003

The North Carolina legislature eliminated Medicaid funding for routine infant circumcision during the 2002 legislative session, effective 1 December 2002.[51] In addition, five other state Medicaid programs also defunded circumcision in 2002: Arizona, effective 1 November 2002; Missouri, effective 1 July 2002; and Montana, effective 1 January 2002.[52-54] In 2003, Utah and Florida also eliminated Medicaid payment for elective circumcisions, bringing the total number of states that do not cover elective circumcisions under Medicaid to twelve.[55-56]

Grass roots efforts in several other states have formed to demand that states eliminate the subsidy of this unnecessary and harmful cultural practice using tax dollars.[57]

REFERENCES

1. North Carolina Medicaid Bulletin. Division of Medical Assistance. (October 2001): p. 6.
2. Council on Scientific Affairs, American Medical Association, Neonatal circumcision. Chicago: American Medical Association, 2000.
3. American Academy of Pediatrics: Task Force on Circumcision. Circumcision policy statement. Pediatrics 1999 Mar;103(3):686-93.
4. The American Academy of Pediatrics and the American College of Obstetricians and Gynecologists. In: Guidelines Perinatal Care, 4th ed. American Academy of Pediatrics, 1997.
5. Wallerstein E. Circumcision: the uniquely American medical enigma. Urologic Clinics of North America 1985 Feb;12(1):123-32.
6. Craig, AL, Cruz, R, Denniston, GC, Svoboda, JS, Travis, JW. Tax Dollar Funding of Medically Unnecessary Circumcision Through Medicaid. International Coalition for Genital Integrity. [Cited 16 March 2001].
   URL: http://www.icgi.org/Medicaid/MedicaidReport.pdf
7. Bell, Dawson. Circumcision may be cut. Detroit Free Press. 12 November 2001.
8. Avery, Sarah. Medicaid won't cover circumcision. Raleigh News and Observer. 31 October 2001.
9. Sheehan, Ruth. Save $200 and shame a poor boy. Raleigh News and Observer. 5 November 2001.
10. Avery, Sarah. Medicaid won't cover circumcision. Raleigh News and Observer. 31 October 2001.
11. Avery, Sarah. Medicaid won't cover circumcision. Raleigh News and Observer. 31 October 2001.
12. Avery, Sarah. Medicaid won't cover circumcision. Raleigh News and Observer. 31 October 2001.
13. Swope, Christopher. Budget Cuts Touch a Nerve. Governing Magazine (January 2002): p. 14.
14. Via phone conversation on 1 November 2001 with editor Kathy Williams.
15. HCIA-Sachs, Inc. Baltimore, Maryland, (800) 568-3282, info@hcia.com.
16. Editor. Close to bone. Raleigh News and Observer. 24 February 2002.

17. Tang, Suk-fong, Ph.D. Medicaid Reimbursement Survey, 2001: 50 States and the District of Columbia. American Academy of Pediatrics, Division of Health Policy Research, 2001.
18. Tang, Suk-fong, Ph.D. Medicaid Reimbursement Survey, 2001: 50 States and the District of Columbia. American Academy of Pediatrics, Division of Health Policy Research, 2001.
19. Craig, AL, Cruz, R, Denniston, GC, Svoboda, JS, Travis, JW. Tax Dollar Funding of Medically Unnecessary Circumcision through Medicaid. International Coalition for Genital Integrity. [cited 16 March 2001].
    URL: http://www.icgi.org/Medicaid/MedicaidReport.pdf
20. As reported by an aide in North Carolina State Senator Howard Lee's office via a phone conversation, 13 December 2001.
21. Mansfield CJ, Hueston WJ, Rudy M. Neonatal circumcision: associated factors and length of hospital stay. J Fam Pract 1995 Oct;41(4):370-6.
22. Mansfield CJ, Hueston WJ, Rudy M. Neonatal circumcision: associated factors and length of hospital stay. J Fam Pract 1995 Oct;41(4):370-6.
23. Adler R, Ottaway S, Gould S. Circumcision: we have heard from the experts; now let's hear from the parents. Pediatrics 2001 Feb;107(2):e20.
24. American Academy of Pediatrics: Task Force on Circumcision. Circumcision policy statement. Pediatrics 1999 Mar;103(3):686-93.
25. Sheehan, Ruth. Save $200 and shame a poor boy. Raleigh News and Observer. 5 November 2001.
26. Bollinger D. (2000) Intact Versus Circumcised: Male Neonatal Genital Ratio in the United States. Circumcision Reference Library (an original online publication), 13 November 2000. http://www.cirp.org/library/statistics/bollinger3/
27. Bonner, Lynn. Medicaid Benefit Restored. Raleigh News and Observer, 17 November 2001.
28. Comment made by Senator Ellie Kinnaird via phone conversation, 6 December 2001.
29. Comment made by Representative Verla Insko via phone conversation, 7 December 2001.
30. E-mail correspondence by North Carolina Representative Fern Shubert, 16 November 2001.
31. E-mail correspondence by North Carolina Senator Fountain Odom, 21 November 2001.
32. E-mail correspondence by North Carolina Senator James Forrester, 28 November 2001.
33. E-mail correspondence by North Carolina Senator Ken Moore, 19 November 2001.
34. E-mail correspondence by North Carolina Senator Virginia Foxx, 28 November 2001.
35. North Carolina General Assembly – Senate, Sequence number 1217/8, HB 231 SCS 6th Edition, 6 December 2001.
36. As reported by an aide in North Carolina State Senator Howard Lee's office via a phone conversation, 13 December 2001.
37. Comment made by Senator Ellie Kinnaird via phone conversation, 6 December 2001.
38. Comment made by aide in Senator Howard Lee's office via phone conversation, 13 December 2001.
39. North Carolina General Assembly – Senate, Sequence number 1217/8, HB 231 SCS 6th Edition, 6 December 2001.
40. North Carolina House of Representatives Roll Call, Sequence number 1493, HB 231 SCS 2, 6 December 2001.
41. Reported by Franklin Freeman via phone conversation, 11 December 2001.
42. Swope, Christopher. Budget cuts touch a nerve. Governing Magazine (January 2002): p. 14.
43. Reporter Lynn Bonner denied request over phone to write a story detailing taxpayer concerns over funding of circumcision on 7 December 2001.
44. Marc Basnight, personal correspondence, 19 December 2001.

45. Avery, Sarah. Study: Dental care lacking with Medicaid. Raleigh News and Observer. 27 December 2001.

46. Wilson, Trish. Tough Choices — Medicaid cuts freeze elder care program, leave relatives scrambling. Raleigh News and Observer. 8 February 2002.

47. Christensen, Rob. States awash in red ink. Raleigh News and Observer. 10 February 2002.

48. O'Connor, Paul. Medicaid has state in stranglehold. The Chapel Hill News. 3 February 2002.

49. Wilson, Trish. Tough Choices —— Medicaid cuts freeze elder care program, leave relatives scrambling. Raleigh News and Observer. 8 February 2002.

50. O'Connor, Paul. Serious crisis. The Chapel Hill News. 10 February 2002.

51. Mike Stobbe. Circumcision funding halted. Charlotte Observer (Charlotte, North Carolina). 21 September 2002.

52. St. John, Stevie. Medicaid to drop practice. The Missourian (Columbia, Missouri). 25 July 2002.

53. Griffiths, Lawn. Arizona rightly ended funds for circumcisions. The East Valley/Scottsdale Tribune (Mesa/Scottsdale). 14 June 2002.

54. McKee, Jennifer. Medicaid cuts announced. The Missoulian (Missoula). 20 December 2002.

55. Jacob Santini. Some health care bills made it, some didn't. Salt Lake Tribune (Saturday, 8 March 2003).

56. Alisa Ulferts. State limits circumcision coverage: Medicaid will no longer cover most of the surgeries in Florida as state officials seek to reduce costs. St. Petersburg Times 1 July 2003. URL: http://www.sptimes.com/2003/07/01/State/State_limits_circumci.shtm

57. Liptak, Adam. Circumcision opponents use legal system and legislatures. New York Times. 23 January 2003. URL:
http://www.nytimes.com/2003/01/23/national/23CIRC.html

Chapter 16

ADOPTION
A Path to Genital Integrity

Gregory J. Hartley, BSc, PE
Director, National Organization of Circumcision Information Resource Centers of Pennsylvania

Abstract: The adoption process presents opportunities for the protection of genital integrity. Two different types of adoption are addressed: domestic (United States) and international. Based on cultural differences, international adoptees are more likely to remain intact. Adoptive parents are often reluctant to circumcise a child past the newborn stage, under the belief that the procedure is more traumatic than neonatal circumcision. Because many adoptees are of a different racial or ethnic background from the adoptive parents, the impulse to impose circumcision on a child to make him "look like dad" is attenuated. There are many opportunities for to protect intact boys.

Key words: Adoption, circumcision, foreskin

1.   INTRODUCTION

Compared to biological parenting, adoption often provides children with a greater chance to be allowed the dignity of remaining physically intact. The promotion of bodily integrity through adoption is a timely issue that deserves attention from human rights activists. Adoption of children has increased in recent years. Although there is no comprehensive information available for domestic adoption,[1] growing numbers of children are being adopted from outside the US. In the US, adopted children often have a greater chance of keeping their genitalia intact than children who are biologically related to their parents. The process of building a family through adoption, although similar in many ways to biological birth, involves some distinct differences that can be utilized to protect a child's genital integrity.

Flesh and Blood, Edited by Denniston et al.
Kluwer Academic/Plenum Publishers, New York 2004

This paper assumes the inherent right of self-determination and genital integrity for all children. The benefits of intact genitalia or the harm of involuntary genital cutting are not discussed in detail, as these topics are documented elsewhere.[2-3]

My interest in this subject is personal. In late 1997, my wife Karen and I were going through the process of adopting a child from Russia. I had done some reading and realized that non-religious circumcision was virtually unheard of in Russia. My wife and I felt very fortunate that our son was intact, and we resolved to protect his right to remain that way. Because I was indebted to those who had helped to educate me about genital integrity, I volunteered to present a circumcision lecture at the placement agency that facilitated our son's adoption. My lecture became part of the required training, for prospective parents, given by that agency.

2.   DOMESTIC (US) AND INTERNATIONAL ADOPTION

Two very different types of adoption are discussed in this paper: domestic (referring to adoption of children within the US) and international (children born outside the US). The characteristics of these two types will be discussed throughout the sections of this paper, but they are all based on one essential element: the circumcision decision made by the birthmother. This decision is often made in favor of genital integrity.

Although this paper deals primarily with the adoption of infants, there were over a half million children of all ages in domestic foster care in 1999.[4] Some of these children may not have been circumcised as infants. Just as a biological parent or an adoption agency should not circumcise children, foster children should not be circumcised at the whim of foster parents. No child should be subjected to the physical pain and trauma inherent in genital cutting at the behest of those whom he is learning to trust. Fortunately, most agencies do not permit foster parents to authorize elective surgeries such as circumcision.

In the US, approximately sixty percent of newborn males are circumcised. Therefore, one can expect this percentage to apply to prospective adoptee male infants as well. There are no specific statistics for adoptee circumcision. In most domestic adoptions, the birthmother has sole control of the infant's medical care until the child is discharged from the hospital or birthing center. Upon discharge, a medical power-of-attorney is typically granted to the prospective adoptive parents, who then have legal authority to make medical decisions for the child until the adoption is final.[5] Alternately, the prospective adoptive parents can discuss the issue of circumcision with the birthmother, who may defer to their wishes.[6] The parties may agree that the child should be permitted to remain intact.

Compared to domestic adoptees, children adopted from outside the US (international adoptees) have a much better chance of remaining intact. The process is very different because the child typically resides in an orphanage or baby home when the adoption process begins. The birthmother is not typically involved in any medical decisions for the child. Additionally, in most countries outside the US, non-religious neonatal circumcision is rarely performed. The child must often wait a significant amount of time before he is eligible for adoption. Therefore, most adoptees are beyond the newborn stage. As described later in this paper, these aspects of international adoption work in favor of genital integrity.

3. CULTURAL ISSUES

Although both birthparents are sometimes involved in making a child available for adoption, it is more typically the case that only the birthmother is involved.

The birthmother's cultural conditioning can significantly influence her decision about circumcision for the prospective adoptee. Sometimes, an involved birthfather can be a factor in this decision. Parents and friends of the birthmother, birthfather, and prospective adoptive parents may also influence the child's fate. These factors may promote genital integrity in cultures where circumcision is rare, but they can work against the child's rights in the US. Birthmothers may decide to circumcise their prospective adoptee based on habit or a perceived cultural expectation of the adoptive parents. Some parents mistakenly believe that a child's birth process is not fully complete until a circumcision is performed. Like many Americans, they take it for granted that the procedure will be done by the hospital as part of the delivery.

The cultural norms and concerns of the birthmother can also work in support of bodily integrity. Since she will not be responsible for the child's long-term care, the birthmother may not give any thought to the typical rationalizations for circumcision. She will not need to deal with any perceived "social issues" of the child. She may also feel that this decision should be left to the adoptive parents.

In the US, it is common for a circumcised father to insist that his newborn son be circumcised for no other reason than to make the son "look like dad." This impulse is attenuated in circumcised adoptive fathers. The race, ethnicity, or physical appearance of the adoptee is sometimes quite different from that of the parents. Consequently, these more visible differences often mitigate any parental concern for similar genitalia.

In contrast to domestic adoption, international adoption offers a much better chance for a child to maintain his genital integrity. During the past few years, adoption of orphans from countries outside the US has steadily increased, as shown in Figure 1.[7-9]

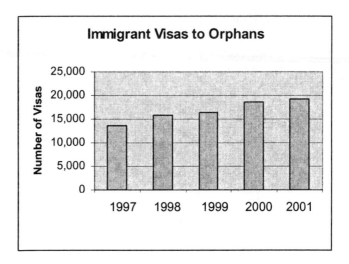

Figure 1: Numbers of Annual Immigrant Visas to Orphans (1997 – 2001)

Countries of origin for most international adoptees have no tradition of neonatal circumcision. From 1997 to 1999, the US issued immigrant visas to orphans, as shown in Table 1.[10] Non-religious circumcision of newborns is essentially nonexistent in the countries listed in this table.

Table 1. Number of Immigrant Visas issued to Orphans coming to the United States

(1997-1999)

Country	Number of Visas
Russia	12,655
China	11,904
South Korea	5,491
Guatemala	2,701
Romania	1,516
Vietnam	603
Other	10,560
Total	45,430

South Korea stands out as a slight anomaly. Although circumcision in this Asian country is widespread, only a small percentage of the procedures are performed during the neonatal period. The median age for circumcision in South Korea is twelve, and fewer than ten percent of infants are circumcised in the neonatal period.[11] Since almost half of all international adoptees are under one year of age, and almost ninety percent are under four,[12] the majority of South Korean children can be assumed to possess intact genitalia when they are adopted. Despite the high overall circumcision rate in South Korea, these children also have a better chance for genital integrity than domestic adoptees.

For many adoptive parents of children born outside the US, the child's cultural identity has some influence on the way in which the child is raised. In my interactions with parents of international adoptees, many express a desire to preserve some aspects of their child's cultural identity. Sometimes this includes maintaining the child's genital integrity, prevalent in most countries outside the US. As an adoptee matures, he or she may begin to explore the culture of their birthplace. In cases where there is a racial difference between the adoptive parents and child, this new identification with the native culture can be strong. Leaving the child intact will allow the child to better relate to his native culture.

4.   CIRCUMCISION PAIN

Typically, concerns about the pain involved in circumcision have little influence on the genital integrity status of domestic adoptees, but pain is usually a significant factor in international adoption. Like many Americans, the birthmother in a domestic case is usually not familiar with the severe pain and trauma associated with infant circumcision.[13] Many prospective parents of international adoptees, however, give this issue some consideration, based on the common perception that circumcision pain is more severe for an older infant or child. Most children adopted from outside the US are older than domestic adoptees, usually by several months or years.

For most of the prospective adoptive parents in my circumcision lectures, the pain issue was the deciding factor in keeping the child intact. Many parents believe that circumcision is more painful and traumatic for an older child compared to the pain felt by an infant. In terms of physical pain, however, this view is incorrect. During a neonatal circumcision, the foreskin must be forcibly torn from the glans penis before it can be excised because, at birth, the glans and the inner surface of the foreskin are fused[14] The foreskin gradually separates from the glans as the child develops, and it usually is fully retractable by puberty.[15] Therefore, during circumcision of an older child, the foreskin does not need to be torn from the glans, an extremely painful part of the infant circumcision procedure. Furthermore, it is much easier to administer pain medication to an older child than to an infant. It may also be less traumatic because, unlike an infant, the older child may be somewhat aware of what is about to happen. On the other hand, the older child's increased awareness may increase the level of trauma because the child is understandably horrified by the idea of having part of his penis amputated.

Although the physical pain of circumcision suffered by an older child is arguably less severe than an infant's pain, the procedure is extremely traumatic at any age for a child. Goldman discusses the pain and trauma associated with the circumcision of older children.[16] The general issue of pain and trauma should be reinforced to parents rather than the specific degree of pain involved for an infant compared to an older child. Many adoptive parents are careful about protecting their child from any trauma. This is especially true for international adoptees, who may have endured difficult circumstances during infancy. The adoptive parents do not want the child's first memory of his new family to be associated with an extremely painful procedure.

Finally, it is much easier to care for a genitally intact child. The post-operative treatment following circumcision involves frequent dressing changes and pushing back the foreskin remnant to prevent adhesions. As discussed in the next section, "Leave it alone" is good advice for an intact child.

5.   OPPORTUNITIES FOR ACTIVISM

During the last decade, adoption of children from countries outside the US has been increasing, due in part to the collapse of communist governments in Russia and Eastern Europe, and to the opening of these societies to Western influence. Some of these countries have experienced difficult economic conditions during the transition to a market-based economy. These conditions contribute to increased abandonment of newborns by birthmothers, who are often unmarried and cannot support a child. The steady growth in international adoption is illustrated in Figure 1.

Despite the increasing prevalence of international adoption, the *Hague Convention on Intercountry Adoption* does not contain a provision that respects the genital integrity of children.[17] This multilateral treaty was adopted on 29 May 1993 at The Hague and has been signed by the US and ratified by Congress. Implementation will occur only after the Immigration and Naturalization Service and the Department of State publish regulations in the *Federal Register*, which is expected within the next two years.[18] A worthy goal for human rights activists would be the development of a regulation that protects the child's inalienable right to genital integrity.

The Joint Council on International Child Services (JCICS) is the oldest and largest affiliation of licensed nonprofit international adoption agencies in the world.[19] JCICS holds annual conferences dealing with many issues related to international adoption. According to a regular attendee, this body has not specifically addressed the issue of genital integrity for adoptees.[20]

The care of intact children is an area of the adoption process that requires special focus, primarily in the training of prospective adoptive parents. Adoption agencies require completion of a training program for their clients. The training is required prior to finalizing the adoption. These programs, which are not necessarily consistent between agencies, cover a wide range of subjects and are meant to educate parents on the adoption process and to cope with any potential problems. When my wife and I attended classes given by the agency that facilitated the adoption of our son, the subject of circumcision was never mentioned. Based on my discussions with several adoptive parents and adoption agencies, issues related to circumcision are not usually covered during this training.

I persuaded the agency to include a circumcision lecture as part of the required prospective parent training. When I presented my lecture, I discussed the proper method of care of intact infants. [21] The program coordinator, also an adoptive parent, appeared to be very distressed during my talk. She later told me that she had been attempting forced retraction of her infant son during his bath, which is inconsistent with guidance from the American Academy of Pediatrics.[22]

> Care of the uncircumcised boy is quite easy. "Leave it alone" is good advice. External washing and rinsing on a daily basis is all that is required. Do not retract the foreskin in an infant, as it is almost always attached to the glans. Forcing the foreskin back may harm the penis, causing pain, bleeding, and possible adhesions. The natural separation of the foreskin from the glans may take many years. After puberty, the adult male learns to retract the foreskin and cleanse under it on a daily basis.

The child had apparently complained that foreskin retraction bothered him, but she, like many doctors, mistakenly believed that it was necessary. This example illustrates the need for a factual discussion of intact care during pre-adoption training. Premature retraction of the foreskin can result in a myriad of problems.[23]

Part of this problem is related to the decision process used by adoptive parents of children born overseas. Unlike many US birthparents who respect their son's genital integrity after learning about the circumcision problem, parents of international adoptees may decide to keep their son intact solely to avoid trauma, as discussed above. These parents may not have reached their decision through detailed research on the subject. Therefore, they may not fully understand all the issues related to circumcision or the proper care of intact genitalia.

6. CONCLUSION

There is a need to draw attention to the adoption process as it relates to the promotion of genital integrity, especially in the area of international adoption. Adoption is a process where the inherent right of bodily integrity for all children can and should be emphasized. Part of this advocacy effort should include prospective parent training with a focus on the reasons for keeping children intact and education about the proper care of intact genitalia. Other aspects include the establishment of government regulations and adoption agency guidelines that respect a child's right to bodily integrity.

ACKNOWLEDGEMENTS

I would like to acknowledge the input of my fellow adoptive parent, Albert Fields, Director of the Philadelphia center of NOCIRC-Pennsylvania. I especially recognize the contribution of my wife Karen. This paper (and my activism) would not be possible without her encouragement and support.

REFERENCES

1. National Adoption Information Clearinghouse, Adoption Statistics: Table of Contents. http://www.calib.com/naic/stats/index.htm
2. This reference and the following one are good starting points to explore the benefits of genital integrity and the harm of circumcision. National Organization of Circumcision Information Resource Centers www.nocirc.org
3. Circumcision Information and Resources Page www.cirp.org
4. US Dept. Health & Human Services, Administration for Children and Families, Adoption and Foster Care Analysis and Reporting System (ACFARS) data for FY 1999.
5. Petrillo MA. Personal communication.
6. Lesko D. Personal communication.
7. National Adoption Information Clearinghouse, Intercountry Adoption. http://www.calib.com/naic/pubs/s_inter.htm
8. US Department of State, The Bureau of Consular Affairs. http://travel.state.gov/orphan_numbers.html
9. Snider J. USA Today (26 February 2002): p. D7
10. National Adoption Information Clearinghouse, Intercountry Adoption.

http://www.calib.com/naic/pubs/s_inter.htm

11. Pang MG, Kim SC, Kim DS. Male circumcision in South Korea: history, statistics, and the role of doctors in creating a circumcision rate of over 100%. In: Denniston GC, Hodges FM, Milos MF (eds). Understanding Circumcision: A Multi-Disciplinary Approach to a Multi-Dimensional Problem. New York: Kluwer Academic Publishers, 2001. pp. 61-81.

12. National Adoption Information Clearinghouse, Intercountry Adoption.
http://www.calib.com/naic/pubs/s_inter.htm

13. Goldman R. Circumcision: The Hidden Trauma. Boston: Vanguard Publishers, 1997. pp. 20-4.

14. Cold CJ, Taylor JR. The prepuce. BJU Int. 1999 Jan;83 Suppl 1:34-44.

15. CIRP: Normal development of the prepuce: Birth through age 18
www.cirp.org/library/normal/

16. Goldman R. Circumcision: The Hidden Trauma. Boston: Vanguard Publishers, 1997. pp. 101-2.

17. Hague Convention on Intercountry Adoption
http://travel.state.gov/adoption_info_sheet.html

18. The Intercountry Adoption Act of 2000
http://www.ins.usdoj.gov/graphics/publicaffairs/factsheets/adoption.htm

19. Joint Council on International Child Services http://www.jcics.org/mission.html

20. Springer S. Personal communication.

21. NOCIRC Information Series, Pamphlet 4. Answers to Your Questions About Your Son's Intact Penis. http://www.nocirc.org/publish/pam4.html

22. American Academy of Pediatrics pamphlet. Newborns: Care of the Uncircumcised Penis – Guidelines for Parents. 1990.

23. NOCIRC Information Series, Pamphlet 6. Answers to Your Questions about Premature (Forced) Retraction of Your Young Son's Foreskin.
http://www.nocirc.org/publish/pam6.html

Chapter 17

GEORGE WALD
A Personal Reminiscence of a Nobel Laureate

Van Lewis
Assistant to the President, Students for Genital Integrity, Florida State University

Abstract: This paper is a personal reminiscence of the Harvard biology professor and Nobel laureate George Wald. It presents a history of Wald's position against circumcision and an account of Wald's efforts to publish a critique of circumcision from 1975 until his death in 1997.

Key words: Nobel Prize, George Wald, Harvard University, circumcision, human rights

1.   INTRODUCTION

The movement to secure the right to bodily integrity for all people has strong support from some of the world's finest scientists. It was with great joy that I discovered the "Ashley Montagu Resolution to End the Genital Mutilation of Children Worldwide — A Petition to the World Court, The Hague," written by James W. Prescott, PhD, and adopted in 1996 by the General Assembly of the Fourth International Symposium on Sexual Mutilations in Lausanne, Switzerland. I soon learned that Nobel laureate biologist, Francis Crick, co-discoverer of the structure of the DNA molecule and winner of the 1962 Nobel Prize in Physiology or Medicine, had endorsed this important human rights resolution in 1995.

George Wald (1906-1997), a child of immigrant New York Jewish parents, beloved Harvard biology professor, and an important twentieth-century social activist for peace and justice, also worked to defend the right of all children, male and female, to genital integrity. In 1975, Wald wrote and offered for publication in *The New Yorker* an essay entitled "Circumcision." He may, therefore, have been the first Nobel laureate to work to protect children from genital mutilation.

Flesh and Blood, Edited by Denniston et al.
Kluwer Academic/Plenum Publishers, New York 2004

2.   MEETING GEORGE WALD

I first learned about Wald in my freshman dormitory room at Harvard in September 1961. Some upstart Harvard students had been grading their professors and publishing this effrontery as the "Confidential Guide." It was our "Bible" in our twice-yearly search for courses. I learned two important things from the guide. First, "Get a freshman seminar if you can," which I was very fortunate to do with a wonderful Greek anthropologist, Dr. Dorothy Lee; and second, "Don't you dare leave Harvard without getting to know George Wald. The best way to begin is to take his course, Natural Sciences 5, one of Harvard's best."

I accepted the wisdom of my elders — unusual for me — and enrolled. Wald's course, "The Nature of Living Things," was much more than an introductory biology course. It was a tour of the then known physical universe with a tour guide who would soon be awarded the 1967 Nobel Prize for his discovery of Vitamin A in the retina of the eye and how it works with light to produce the molecular and energetic basis of vision. A top research scientist, Wald was later declared by *Time* magazine one of America's ten best teachers.

Wald loved teaching freshmen because, as he said, "their minds are still fresh." We loved Wald because he embodied for us what Albert Schweitzer called "reverence for life," and he made it clear to us that "life" for him included us, individually.

George included in his reverence the entire scientifically knowable world, not just the biological life within it. The nonliving universe was as much to be studied, understood, appreciated, and revered as biological life, which, for him as an evolutionist, had arisen within this amazing and lawful structure and process we know as physical reality. We are, he believed, intrinsic to the universe, and it to us. "We're home here," he taught us.

Wald was loved by students at Harvard because he was not only an exciting teacher and revealer of the nature of reality as seen in some ways so clearly and so exquisitely by science but also a deeply humane, gentle, strong, loving, vital, good-humored, intelligent, and articulate man.

Wald's professional life, in addition to the teaching he loved so much, was one dedicated to the process of asking scientific questions and finding verifiable scientific answers. He told us that answers are relatively easy to come by; that the really difficult but exciting and important part — not just of science but of life — is sensing what questions are important to ask in the first place and figuring out how to ask them intelligently so that the correct answers come out as a matter of course.

3.   WALD'S NOBEL PRIZE

Let me take you into the heart of his scientific world for a moment. Here is a short paragraph from the Nobel presentation speech to Wald and his fellow Nobel laureates in 1967:

> Professor Granit, Professor Hartline, Professor Wald. Your discoveries have deepened our insight into the nature of the subtle processes in the eye which form the basis of our ability to perceive light and to distinguish brightness, color, form and movement. They have also proved to be of paramount importance for the understanding of sensory processes in general.[1]

I believe Wald's long and productive research on the eye helped illuminate his deep concern with and writings about consciousness.[2]

In the same presentation speech, we read:

> Professor Wald. With a deep biological insight and a great biochemical skill you have successfully identified visual pigments and their precursors. As a byproduct you were able to describe the absorption spectra of the different types of cones serving colour vision. Your most important discovery of the primary molecular reaction to light in the eye represents a dramatic advance in vision since it plays the role of a trigger in the photoreceptors of all living animals.

Wald began his Nobel acceptance speech by talking about questions and answers:

> I have often had cause to feel that my hands are cleverer than my head. That is a crude way of characterizing the dialectics of experimentation. When it is going well it is like a quiet conversation with Nature. One asks a question and gets an answer; then asks the next question and gets the next answer. An experiment is a device to make Nature speak intelligibly. After that one has only to listen.[3]

4.   QUESTIONS AND ANSWERS ABOUT CIRCUMCISION

The questions I had asked myself at Harvard and afterward about the anthropology, biology, history, mythology, religion, psychology, and psychopathology underlying human genital mutilations had been followed by some frequently disturbing but — with hindsight — inevitable answers. Often, I wished I had never asked these questions nor listened to or heard their disturbing answers, but for me there was no turning back to the ignorant bliss of earlier years.

By 1969, I was becoming frustrated in my search for the right questions. I had reached a plateau in my understanding and felt that I was blocked in making further internal progress, perhaps because I was not sharing the bad news I had discovered. Withholding important information from others, I sensed that I might also be unconsciously withholding further important information about genital mutilation from myself.

I decided to make my hard-won (if so far incomplete) answers public in Tallahassee by staging an anti-circumcision protest in front of Tallahassee Memorial Hospital. For this effrontery, my brother, Ben, and I were arrested and jailed for several hours on 17 December 1970.

Shortly afterward, I asked myself, "What would it feel like if I had never been circumcised? What would it feel like to have a foreskin where it belongs?" I imagined that the foreskin would be warm flesh enclosing and protecting my glans penis. The foreskin seemed to me, at that moment, to be a male "vagina."

It occurred to me that the doctor who circumcised me in 1943 — along with every other circumciser who, for millennia, has been compelled to cut boys' foreskins off— may have subconsciously regarded the male foreskin as somehow "feminine." The gender identity anxieties and homophobia underlying the phenomenon of circumcision had suddenly become apparent to me.

I felt I had asked another important question and received another answer I had been seeking for the nine puzzling years since Harvard.

5.   WALD'S INTRODUCTION TO THE CIRCUMCISION QUESTION

Four years later, in February 1975, Wald was invited to Florida State University in Tallahassee to give a lecture about life. I attended and also went to the discussion and the reception afterwards with my mother, wife, and baby daughter. I asked Wald if I could take him to the airport when he was ready to go, and he agreed. I knew what question I had to ask him.

"George, have you every thought much about circumcision — from a biological point of view?" His eyes grew big. He was surprised by my question, I think, not because I had asked it, but because he — a Nobel laureate Harvard biologist who had spent his scientific career studying a human sensory system in molecular detail — never had. Not my question, but his own answer shocked him. "No," he said. "I never have. I'll have to go home and do that."

On the way to the airport, I related to him the history of my interest in the problem of genital mutilations, from my college days, my plateau, the block

I had reached by 1969 in my own efforts at understanding, my consequent decision to go public with my protest, and the arrest.

We arrived at the airport and discovered that his plane was delayed. I had him to myself in the Tallahassee airport for two hours. We continued our conversation. In Wald's account of our discussion later that year, he wrote, "Suddenly he said something that shook me." I told him about my reward for the jailing, the surprising insight about finding a "female" sex organ on the penis. "My God!" he exclaimed, "that's wonderful! Because we've always been told that the clitoris is the male element in a female!" Then he told me about the Dogon, an African tribe that practices both male and female genital mutilation. His plane arrived and I had to let him go.

6. THE ESSAY

Six months later, Wald sent me a typewritten manuscript entitled "Circumcision." Here, in my own shaking hands was an unpublished, highly enlightening essay by a Nobel laureate and a Harvard biologist on a deeply mysterious and ancient subject of great concern to me. I read it with growing amazement.

In 1971, shortly after my arrest, the American Academy of Pediatrics had issued a statement on circumcision, declaring, "There are no valid medical indications for circumcision in the neonatal period."[4] Young and naive as I was, I assumed that, "The adults are going to take care of this medical quackery! I don't have to go to jail any more! The doctors are going to clean up their own mess. In two years, five at the outside, this will all be over!" And now, after reading Wald's manuscript, I could confirm these beliefs by adding, "And if the doctors have difficulties, the Noble laureates are going to help them!"

As it turned out, these ideas were hopelessly naïve. I had sensed it while in jail, but I really did not appreciate the depth and power of circumcision madness in America.

Since the mid 1970s, tens of millions of American men have been senselessly mutilated as infants by American medical "professionals" who are obviously more concerned with protecting their own income, assets, and privileges than they are with protecting their patients' health, bodily integrity, human rights, and very lives. I believe today just as strongly as I did in 1970, when I was arrested for saying so in public, that circumcisers are sex criminals. The mounting evidence supporting this allegation is so strong, that I am today even more motivated than I was in 1970 to protect males from this abuse.

I took detailed notes on Wald's essay and wrote a long letter back to him expressing my deep appreciation for his brilliant work on the subject and offering many detailed observations about what he had written.

Shortly thereafter, Wald informed me that he had submitted a revised and expanded version of the essay to William Shawn, the editor of *The New Yorker*. Shawn had already published several important essays by Wald. In his cover letter to Shawn, dated 18 August 1975, Wald wrote:

> I have been absorbed all summer in writing the enclosed paper. The beginning of it will tell you how that happened. Gradually I realized that I was writing it for you. I don't know how strange you will find that; but I think that *The New Yorker* has the weight and depth and the readership that I want most to reach and that will most respond. If it jumps off from there it will go far.
>
> The subject has its fascinations of many kinds — social, theological, anthropological, deeply personal; but this essay is trying also to meet a problem, it takes a position. The medical literature turned anti-circumcision ten years ago, but almost none of that has filtered through to the mothers. Perhaps this paper will do that job. There will be plenty of flak.[5]

On 8 September 1975, Shawn replied:

> Broad as our range may be, this subject seems somehow beyond it. What you have to say is, as always, important and sounds right. We are most grateful to you for letting us consider this. I hope that all is well with you.[6]

Wald later told me privately that *The New Yorker* had found his essay "too radical."

In June, 2000, I contacted an editor at *The New Yorker* to obtain more information about Shawn's rejection of Wald's paper. A knowledgeable editor replied:

> I am not at all surprised that Shawn turned it down. The reason, I'm sure, is that he was incredibly queasy about anything involving bodily functions and/or private parts. He wouldn't have even allowed the word 'foreskin' into the magazine, let alone publish an entire article about the cutting off of same.[7]

Shawn was unmoved by the important fact that the essay had been written by a man who was a Noble laureate, a Harvard professor, a highly regarded public figure, an author, a friend, and a Jew. Shawn appears to have been as much a prisoner of genital mutilation as the nation he lived in. Was he afraid of the controversy that both Wald and he knew would erupt if he dared publish this revolutionary material?

In his essay, Wald wrote, "I shall probably not be forgiven this essay." Shawn's refusal to publish Wald's essay was hardly surprising, given his position. Shawn surely knew that he would not have been forgiven either, and he did not enjoy the job security Wald received with his tenured position at Harvard.

Wald was in many ways ahead of his time. When he wrote the essay in 1975, doctors were still regarded almost as gods, and the rate of routine neonatal circumcision in the United States was not only rapidly rising but had already surpassed the ninety-percent mark. The country was engulfed by a tidal wave of institutionalized and banalized surgical reduction of male genitalia.

Ironically, even though it was a common medical procedure, discussing circumcision was deeply taboo, as my jail time had proved. Almost no one wanted to discuss it or allow anyone else to discuss it. This remains just as true in American society today.

As difficult as it would have been for the average American to confront the horror of cutting off the end of a baby's penis, the fact that doctors were behind the campaign gave Americans the false assurance that "everything was all right." The idea that anyone — let alone a Jewish Nobel laureate — might question this trend was simply unthinkable and certainly would have been unacceptable to most Americans. Circumcision depends for its survival on secrecy and public ignorance. As such, circumcisers work hard to make discussion of circumcision taboo.

Whatever the personal feelings of William Shawn, his rejection of an article penned by a world-famous and much loved Harvard biology professor and Nobel laureate was an act of censorship that prevented *The New Yorker* from publishing what certainly would have been an unpopular article in many quarters and prevented the educated, affluent, and influential readers of the magazine from being exposed, in a dramatic way, to ideas that threatened to foment discussion and much-needed debate about America's mistaken acceptance of medicalized genital mutilation in the nineteenth and twentieth centuries.

The New Yorker's censoring of Wald's article also certainly delayed the day when American boys will be free from this medically unjustified criminal assault on and mutilation of their sex organs. This delay has denied a normal sex life to everyone affected and has killed many innocent male babies as well.

In the early 1990s while in Cambridge, Wald mentioned to me that he was serving on the advisory board of a "local Jewish anti-circumcision group." At the time, I was unaware that there was a significant national and international movement against male genital mutilation and, much to my current regret, failed to realize the importance of what he was telling me.

On 5 April 2002, after my presentation of some of this material to the Seventh International Symposium on Human Rights and Modern Society in Washington, D.C., Ronald Goldman, Director of the Circumcision Resource Center (CRC) in Boston,[8] informed me that Wald had served on CRC's professional Advisory board from 22 December 1992, until his death in April 1997. Goldman's letter welcoming Wald to CRC's advisory board wished George well in his continuing efforts to get his essay published.

Wald sought a publisher for "Circumcision" for over two decades, but never found one. The essay remains unpublished today, but Wald insured its survival by depositing a copy of his final version among his extensive papers in the Harvard Archives where it rests today, still ignored — no, still deliberately censored — by a nation even more urgently in need of Wald's wisdom today than when Wald wrote the essay over a quarter-century ago.

I continue to hope that some day the essay itself will be published in complete form, just as Wald wrote it and just as he purposefully left it for the world. It is a magnificent and historic document. One day, the world will know it and revere Wald for it.

7.   AFTERTHOUGHTS

Wald's arguments against circumcision were tailored to the audience he hoped to reach through *The New Yorker*. It is to be expected that his discussion of the issue may seem now, nearly three decades later, somewhat dated and naïve in places, but even though it was written in an era marred by profound medical arrogance and ignorance, Wald's essay broke many cultural and intellectual boundaries.

Despite his parents' cultural background (positive elements of which he rightly cherished), Wald had the intelligence and strength to study the subject of circumcision objectively and carefully even though he was introduced to the issue in a chance conversation. He differentiated the past (including the long human past, distant ancestors', his family's past, and his own past) from clear present responsibilities and from requirements of the human future. In so doing, he arrived at the correct answer to the simple question I had asked him on the way to the airport.

I think that one of the important reasons that Wald was able to understand the issue of circumcision so well and so quickly was that he had spent his scientific career studying the human visual sense organ system in exquisite detail. When I asked him to move the focus of his scientific attention from visual perception to genital and cultural perception, he was able to do so quickly and competently. He had good preparation for it. His long and productive research on the eye helped him later to think more clearly than most in 1975 about the biological importance of normal nerve impulses generated in the male prepuce. Both interests — the eye and the "sexual eye"[9] — helped illuminate his deep concern with consciousness.[10]

I last saw Wald in 1995. "I've finally gotten really old, Van," he said. "Congratulations, George," I replied. He would be ninety in a few months and had lived in every decade of the twentieth century.

Wald died in 1997. To my knowledge, he was the first Nobel laureate to demonstrate the courage and intellectual integrity necessary to formulate a clear and powerful critique of circumcision. May he not be the last!

REFERENCES

1. http://www.nobel.se/medicine/laureates/1967/press.html
2. http://oasis.harvard.edu/html/hua02000frames.html
3. http://www.nobel.se/medicine/laureates/1967/wald-lecture.pdf
4. American Academy of Pediatrics, Committee on Fetus and Newborn. *Standards and Recommendation for Hospital Care of Newborn infants.* 5th ed. Evanston, IL: American Academy of Pediatrics, 1971. p. 110.
5. Wald's letter to William Shawn in Wald's papers in the Harvard Archives. See http://oasis.harvard.edu/html/hua02000frames.html for an extensive listing of these materials.
6. Letter from William Shawn to George Wald in Wald's papers in the Harvard Archives.
7. Private Correspondence, 10 July 2001.
8. http://circumcision.org
9. See http://research.cirp.org
10. See http://oasis.harvard.edu/html/hua02000frames.html

Appendix

1. ORGANIZATIONS

Association Contre la Mutilation des Enfants (A.M.E.). Boite Postale 220, 92108 Boulogne Cedex, France. http://pages.pratique.fr/~ame1/

Circumcision Information Australia. http://www.circinfo.org/

Circumcision Resource Center. Ronald Goldman, PhD. PO Box 232, Boston, Massachusetts, 02133 USA. Tel: 617-523-0088. http://www.circumcision.org/

Doctors Opposing Circumcision (D.O.C.). George Denniston, MD, MPH. 2442 NW Market Street #42, Seattle, WA 98107 USA. Tel: 360-385-1882. Fax: 360-385-1965
. http://weber.u.washington.edu/~gcd/DOC/

Equality Now. Jessica Neuwirth, President. Post Office Box 20646, Columbus Circle Station, New York, NY 10023. Tel: 212-586-0906. Fax: 212-586-1611.

Foundation for Women's Health Research and Development (FORWARD). Adwoa Kluvitse. 40 Eastbourne Terrace, London W2 3QR. Tel: 0171-926-6300. Fax: 0171-725-2796

Inter-African Committee. Berhane Ros-Work, President. 147 rue de Lausanne, CH-1202 Geneva, Switzerland. Tel: 22-731-2420. Fax: 22-738-1823

International Centre for Reproductive Health. Els Leye, FGM Project Coordinator. Ghent University, De Pintelaan 185 P3, 9000 Ghent, Belgium. Tel: +32-9 240.35.64. Fax: +32-9 240.38.67

London Black Women's Health Action Project. Shamis Dirir. Cornwall Avenue Community Centre, First Floor, 1 Cornwall Avenue. London E2 0HW United Kingdom. Tel: 181-980-3503. Fax: 181-980-6314

National Organization of Circumcision Information Resource Centers (NOCIRC) [International Headquarters] Marilyn Fayre Milos, RN, Executive Dirrector. PO Box 2512, San Anselmo, CA 94979-2512. USA.   Tel: 415-488-9883.   Fax: 415-488-9660. http://www.nocirc.org/

National Organization to Halt the Abuse and Routine Mutilation of Males (NOHARMM). Tim Hammond. http://www.noharmm.org/

National Organization of Restoring Men (NORM) International Headquarters. R. Wayne Griffiths, MS, Med, 3505 Northwood Drive, Suite 209, Concord, CA 94520-4506 USA. Tel: 510-827-4066. Fax: 510-827-4119. http://www.norm.org/.

NORM-UK. John P. Warren, MB. Chairman. PO Box 71. Stone, Staffordshire, ST15 0SF, United Kingdom. Tel/Fax: 01785-814-044. http://www.norm-uk.co.uk/

Nurses for the Rights of the Child. Mary Conant, RN, Betty Katz Sperlich, RN, Mary-Rose Booker, RN. 369 Montezuma #354, Santa FE, New Mexico 87501. Tel: 505-989-7377. http://www. cirp.org/nrc/

Rainb♀. Nahid Toubia, MD. 915 Broadway, Suite 1109, New York, NY, 10010-7108 USA. Tel: 212-477-3318. Fax: 212-477-4154

Terres des Femmes. Marion Hulverscheidt, Petra Schnull. Kreuzbergring 10, D-37075 Gottingen, Germany.

2.   WORLD WIDE WEB SITES

Alliance for Transforming the Lives of Children
www.atlc.org/

Association Contre la Mutilation des Enfants (French)
http://pages.pratique.fr/~ame1/

Attorneys for the Rights of the Child
www.arclaw.org/

Birth Psychology
www.birthpsychology.com/birthscene/circ.html

BoysToo.com (Official Website of NOCIRC of North Dakota)

www.boystoo.com

The Circumcision Information and Resource Pages
www.cirp.org/

Circumcision Information Resource Center (Montreal, Canada)
www.infocirc.org/index-e.htm

Circumcision Resource Center (Boston, Massachusetts)
www.circumcision.org/

D.O.C. (Doctors Opposing Circumcision)
www.doctorsopposingcircumcision.org

Female Genital Mutilation Research Home Page
www.fgmnetwork.org/

In Memory of the Sexually Mutilated Child (John A. Erickson)
www.datasync.com/SexuallyMutilatedChild/

International Coalition for Genital Integrity
www.icgi.org/

Intersex Society of North America Home Page
www.isna.org/

Jews Against Circumcision

National Organization of Circumcision Information Resource Centers
www.nocirc.org/

National Organization to Halt the Abuse and Routine Mutilation of Males
www.noharmm.org/

National Organization of Restoring Men (NORM)
www.norm.org/

NORM-UK (Great Britain)
www.norm-uk.org/

Students for Genital Integrity
www.studentsforgenitalintegrity.org/

3.   BOOKS

Sami A. Aldeeb Abu-Sahlieh. *Male and Female Circumcision Among Jews, Christians and Muslims: religious debate.* Beirut, Lebanon: Riad El-Rayyes Books. 2000.

Sami A. Aldeeb Abu-Sahlieh. *Circoncision Masculine – Circonsion Femine: Debat Religieux, Medical, Social et Juridique.* Paris: L'Harmattan. 2001.

Jim Bigelow, PhD. *The Joy of Uncircumcising!* 2nd Edition. Aptos, CA: Hourglass. 1995. [ISBN 0-934061-22-x] www.norm.org

Billy Ray Boyd. *Circumcision Exposed: Rethinking a Medial and Cultural Tradition.* Freedom, CA: The Crossing Press. 1998. [ISBN 0-89594-939-3]

Anne   Briggs. *Circumcision: What Every Parent Should Know.* Charlottesville, VA: Birth & Parenting Publications. 1985. [ISBN 0-9615484-0-1]

George C. Denniston and Marilyn Fayre Milos, eds. *Sexual Mutilations: A Human Tragedy.* New York and London: Plenum Publishing Corporation. 1997. [ISBN 0-3-6-45589-7]

George C. Denniston, Frederick Mansfield Hodges and Marilyn Fayre Milos, eds. *Male and Female Circumcision: Medical, Legal, and Ethical Considerations in Pediatric Practice.* New York: Kluwer Academic/Plenum Publishers.1999. [ISBN 0-306-46131-5]

George C. Denniston, Frederick Mansfield Hodges and Marilyn Fayre Milos, eds. *Understanding Circumcision: A Multi-Disciplinary Approach to a Multi-Dimensional Problem.* New York: Kluwer Academic/Plenum Publishers. 2001.

Efua Dorkenoo. *Cutting The Rose: Female Genital Mutilation: The Practice and its Prevention.* London: Paul & Co Pub Consortium. 1996. [ISBN: 1873194951]

Paul M. Fleiss and Frederick M. Hodges. *What Your Doctor May Not Tell You About Circumcision.* New York: Warner Books. 2001.

Ronald Goldman, PhD. *Circumcision: The Hidden Trauma.* Boston: Vanguard. 1996. [ISBN 0-9644895-3-8]

Ronald Goldman, PhD. *Questioning Circumcision: A Jewish Perspective.* Boston: Vanguard. 1997. [ISBN 0-9644895-6-2]

David L. Gollaher, PhD. *Circumcision: A History of the World's Most Controversial Surgery.* New York: Basic Books. 2000. [ISBN 0-456-04397-6]

Pia Grassivaro Gallo and Franco Viviani, eds. *Female Genital Mutilation: A Public Health Issue Also in Italy.* Proceedings of the 1994

International Symposium on Female Genital Mutilation, May 3rd, 1994, Padua, Italy. Padua: UNIPRESS. 1995.

Gruenbaum, Ellen. The Female Circumcision Controversy. Philadelphia: University of Pennsylvania Press, 2000.

Fran P. Hosken. *The Hosken Report: Genital and Sexual Mutilation of Females.* 4th edition. Lexington, MA: Women's International Network News. 1994. [ISBN 0942096096]]

Hanny Lightfoot-Klein. *Prisoners of Ritual: An Odyssey Into Female Genital Circumcision in Africa.* New York: Harrington Park Press. 1989. [ISBN: 0-918393-68-X]

Hanny Lightfoot-Klein. *Secret Wounds.* Bloomington: 1stBooks, 2002. [ISBN 1-4033-9699-X]

Peggy O'Mara, ed. *Circumcision: The Rest of the Story.* Santa Fe, NM: Mothering.1993. [ISBN 0-914257-11-0]

Thomas J. Ritter, MD, and George C. Denniston, MD. *Doctors Re-examine Circumcision.* 3rd Edition. Aptos, CA: Hourglass. 2002.

Rosemary Romberg. *Circumcision: The Painful Dilemma.* South Hadley, MA: Bergan & Garvey. 1985. [ISBN 0897890736]

Margaret Somerville. *The Ethical Canary: Science, Society and the Human Spirit.* Toronto: Penguin Books. 2000. [ISBN 0 670 89971 2]

Edward Wallerstein. *Circumcision: An American Health Fallacy.* New York. Springer. 1980. [ISBN 0826132405]

Kayla Weiner, PhD, and Arinna Moon, MA., eds. *Jewish Women Speak Out: Expanding the Boundaries of Psychology.* Seattle, WA: Canopy Press. 1995. [ISBN: 0964587807]

4.   VIDEOTAPES/FILMS

The 8th Day. 53 min. VHS. $30ppd in US, $50ppd outside US. Keren Markuze, POB 361425, Los Angeles, CA 90036. Tel: 323-936-6802.

Facing Circumcision: Eight Physicians Tell Their Stories and Reveal the Ethical Dilemmas of Physicians who Circumcise Newborns. Nurses for the Rights of the Child. 20 minutes. VHS. 1998. Nurses for the Rights of the Child. 369 Montezume #354, Santa Fe, New Mexico, 87501. 505-989-7377. www. cirp.org/nrc/

Fire Eyes. Soraya Mire. 60 minutes. sale: 16mm $2,000, video $445, rental: 16mm $300, video $85. Filmakers Library, Inc., 124 East 40th Street, New York, Y 10016 (212-808-4980).

It's a Boy! Victor Schonfeld. 41 minutes. VHS. $295 institutions, $195 individuals, $65 rental. Filmmakers Library, 124 East 40th Street, New York, NY 10016. el: 212:808-4980. Fax: 212-808-4983.

The Nurses of St. Vincent: Saying "No" To Circumcision. Barry Ellsworth. Includes NOHARMM Rally at California Medical Association. VHS. 30 minutes. 29. NOCIRC, POB 2512, San Anselmo, CA 94979.

Whose Body, Whose Rights? Lawrence Dillon and Tim Hammond. 1996. 56 minutes. VHS. Home Sales: Video-Finders, 1-800-343-4727. Educational Sales: $195, Rental $70, Catalogue no. 38342, University of California Extension, Center for Media and Independent Learning, 2000 Center Street, Fourth Floor, Berkeley, CA 94704, 510-642-0460.

5.   NEWSLETTERS

NOCIRC Annual Report. Marilyn Fayre Milos, RN, Editor. NOCIRC. POB 2512. San Anselmo, CA 94979-2512. USA

NOCIRC of Michigan Informant, Norm Cohen, Editor. POB 333, Birmingham, MI 48012

NORM NEWS, David Smith, Editor, Send SASE and Postal Reply Coupon. NORM-UK, POB 71, Stone, Staffordshire ST15 0SF, England.

Contributors

Michel Beauge, MD, is a Medical Doctor and Sexologist, Vice Chairman of the National Union of Sexologists, and the Secretary General of the Group of Western France Sexologists for Advanced Training. Quimper, France.

Charles A. Bonner, JD, is a civil rights, personal injury, and medical malpractice attorney. Sausalito, CA, USA.

Amber Craig, MA, is the Director, NOCIRC of North Carolina and coordinator of the Medicaid Project to bring an end to public funding of non-medically indicated surgery of non-consenting minors. Chapel Hill, NC, USA.

George C. Denniston, MD (Princeton University), MPH (Harvard School of Public Health), is the founder and Director of Doctors Opposing Circumcision (D.O.C.), co-author, *Doctors Re-Examine Circumcision*, co-editor, *Sexual Mutilations: A Human Tragedy, Male and Female Circumcision: Medical, Legal, and Ethical Considerations in Pediatric Practice, and Understanding Circumcision: A Multi-Disciplinary Approach to a Multi-Dimensional Problem,* and Clinical Assistant Professor, Department of Family Medicine, University of Washington. Seattle, WA, USA.

Leonard B. Glick, MD (University of Maryland), PhD (University of Pennsylvania), Professor of Anthropology, Hampshire College, Amherst, MA (retired), is the author of *Abraham's Heirs: Jews and Christians in Medieval Europe* (1999), "Religion and Genocide," in I.W. Charney, ed., *The Widening Circle of Genocide* (1994), and articles on religion and ethnicity. His book, *Circumcision, Jewish Ethnicity, and the Jewish-Christian Encounter*, is in preparation. New Salem, MA, USA.

Ronald Goldman, PhD, psychologist and educator, is the author of *Circumcision: The Hidden Trauma* and *Questioning Circumcision: A Jewish Perspective* and the Executive Director of the Circumcision Resource Center. Boston, MA, USA.

Pia Grassavaro Gallo, PhD, is Associate Professor in general biology, Faculty of Psychology, at the University of Padua. Her research work for the last twenty-seven years has been dedicated to Somali women and to the physical development of children in Somalia. She was invited by the Somali Ministry of Public Health in 1981 to take part in a scientific mission to Somaliland. Her scientific activity in Somalia has received recognition both at national and international levels. Padua, Italy.

Gary Harryman, MA, the coordinator of the National Organization of Restoring Men, Southern California (NORM-SC), is a researcher and author. Topanga, CA, USA.

Gregory J. Hartley, BSc, PE, graduated cum laude from the University of Pittsburgh (Engineering, 1984). He was a civilian instructor at the US Naval Nuclear Propulsion Program and currently works in fleet support. He is Director of NOCIRC of PA and a founding member of NORM-Pittsburgh. Ingomar, PA, USA.

Frederick Mansfield Hodges, DPhil (Oxon), medical historian, is the co-editor of *Male and Female Circumcision: Medical, Legal, and Ethical Considerations in Pediatric Practice* and *Understanding Circumcision: A Multi-Disciplinary Approach to a Multi-Dimensional Problem,* and co-author, *What Your Doctor May Not Tell You About Circumcision: Untold Facts on America's Most Widely Performed – and Most Unnecessary – Surgery,* and the author of many scholarly articles. He currently (2001-2002) holds a post-doctoral research associateship in the Department of History at Yale University.

Yngve Hofvander, MD, pediatrician and Professor, International Child Health, Uppsala University, Sweden, is a consultant to the Swedish International Development Authority, the World Health Organization, and UNICEF. Uppsala, Sweden.

Van Lewis, is the Director, NOCIRC of Florida. Panacea, FL, USA.

Marica Livio, PhD, Department of General Psychology, University of Padua, Italy

David J. Llewellyn, BA, JD, is a practicing attorney at law, representing plaintiffs in wrongful circumcision and other genital injury cases. Atlanta, GA, USA.

Harry Meislahn BA, MBA, magna cum laude graduate in Economics (Harvard), MBA recipient (Harvard Business School), is the Director of NOCIRC of Illinois. Winnetka, IL, USA.

Marilyn Fayre Milos, RN, is the co-founder and Executive Director of the National Organization of Circumcision Information Resource Centers (NOCIRC), coordinator of the International Symposia on Circumcision, Genital Integrity, and Human Rights. editor, *NOCIRC Annual Report*, and co-editor of *Sexual Mutilations: A Human Tragedy, Male and Female Circumcision: Medical, Legal, and Ethical Considerations In Pediatric Practice,* and *Understanding Circumcision: A Multi-Disciplinary Approach To a Multi-Dimensional Problem.* San Anselmo, CA, USA.

Mark D. Reiss, MD, is a retired physician, an active member of a Conservative synagogue, a grandfather, a child's rights activist, and a researcher. San Francisco, CA, USA.

Marianne M. Sarkis, MA, Applied Medical Anthropologist, is the Director of the Female Genital Mutilation Awareness and Education Project of NOCIRC and the originator of the first female genital mutilation web site. Tampa, FL, USA.

J. Steven Svoboda, JD, graduated cum laude from Harvard Law School and now focuses on the areas of civil litigation and human rights. He is the founder and Executive Director of Attorneys for the Rights of the Child (ARC), a non-profit organization addressing the illegality of involuntary genital surgery. Berkeley, CA, USA.

John Taylor, MB, FRCPC, is a pathologist (retired), Health Sciences Centre and University of Manitoba and researcher. His landmark paper, "The prepuce: specialized mucosa of the penis and its loss to circumcision," was published in the B*ritish Journal of Urology* (1996). Winnipeg, Manitoba, Canada.

Franco Viviani, PhD, graduated in biological sciences from the University of Padua, where he is now professor of Psychobiology at both the Faculty of Medicine and of Psychology. In 1986, he directed the film *Somali Schoolgirls Speak*, a documentary on female genital mutilation in Somalia. In 1991, he participated in a field research project on genital mutilation and, that same year, he and Professor Pia Grassivaro Gallo received honorable mention from the Royal Academy of Overseas Science (Belgium). He has organized surveys, research projects, and symposia on female genital mutilation. Padua, Italy.

Index

247